Running & Science

Running & Science

Editors
Jens Bangsbo &
Henrik B. Larsen

Series editor
Jens Bangsbo

Munksgaard

Institute of Exercise and Sport Sciences
University of Copenhagen

Copenhagen 2000

RUNNING & SCIENCE
Copyright © 2001 Institute of Exercise and Sport Sciences,
University of Copenhagen

Editors: Jens Bangsbo & Henrik B. Larsen
Series editor: Jens Bangsbo
Design and layout: Allis Skovbjerg Jepsen
Front page: Robert Delaunay: Løberne, 1926.
Fotos: p. 18, 48, 66, 108, 119: Sports Foto.
p. 84: Sparta Archive.
p. 122, 137, 148: Private.

ISBN 87 16 12349-9

Printed in Denmark 2001.

Institute of Exercise and Sport Sciences
University of Copenhagen
Nørre Allé 51
DK-2200 Copenhagen

Phone: +45 35 32 08 29
Fax: +45 35 32 08 70
e-mail: IFI@ifi.ku.dk
Homepage: www.ifi.ku.dk

Content

Preface

In August 1997 the 2nd "European Congress of Sport and Exercise Science" was held in Copenhagen with more than 800 participants. The scientific programme covered all aspects of exercise and sport sciences with more than 100 invited speakers and 400 presentations. Within the theme "Science and Sport" a number of symposia covered sports from a multidiciplinary perspective. As many people have expressed an interest in this multidisciplinary approach of sport we have decided to produce a series of books on „soccer", „sailing", „running" and „European diversity in sport and physical activity", respectively. We have been fortunate that so many experts have agreed to contribute to the books allowing for an integration of physiological, psychological, historical and social aspects of the sport. Each chapter in the books provides up-to-date knowledge about the topic and includes a high number of references to allow the reader to go further into depth with the subject area. It is anticipated and hoped that the books will be useful for university researchers, teachers and students as well as for interested coaches.

We will like to express our appreciation to the authors and reviewers as well as the editors for their great effort, which has enabled us to produce these informative books.

Jens Bangsbo
Series Editor

Preword

This book gathers a number of disciplines relevant to science of running. A number of chapters focus on the various aspects of performance in running, whereas others deal with how to train to improve performance in running with specific descriptions of the training performed by former top-class runners. The aspect of how to avoid injuries is also thoroughly covered. All chapters provide up-to-date knowledge about running. Any scientific approach has to have its foundation in practical experiences with running and the authors of this book are duly selected by their combined scientific expertise and long-term practical experience with running. Thus, the book is a useful tool for researches, teachers, coaches and runners to understand how to optimise performance in running.

We will take this opportunity to extend our gratitude to the authors and the individuals who have been involved in the reviewing of chapters in this book, Preben K. Pedersen, Jean-René Lacour, Jan Svedenhag, Erik B. Simonsen, A. Lennart Julin, Gustav Schwenk and Michael Kjær.

We hope you will find the book interesting and enjoy your reading.

Jens Bangsbo & Henrik B. Larsen
Editors

List of Editors and Authors

JESPER L. ANDERSEN, Copenhagen Muscle Research Centre, Department of Molecular Muscle Biology, Rigshospitalet, Section 9312, Juliane Mariesvej 20, 1.th., 2100 Copenhagen Ø, Denmark. Telephone: (+45) 3545 6501 Fax: (+45) 3545 6500 E-mail: jla@rh.dk

JENS BANGSBO, Institute of Exercise and Sport Sciences, University of Copenhagen, Universitetsparken 13, 2100 Copenhagen Ø, Denmark. Telephone: (+45) 3532 1623 Fax: (+45) 3532 1600 E-mail: JBangsbo@aki.ku.dk

CARLO CAPELLI, Dipartimento di Scienze e Tecnologie Biomediche, School of Medicine, University of Udine, Via Gervasutta 48, 33100, Udine, Italy. Telephone: (+39) 432 520188 Fax: (+39) 432 600828 E-mail:carlo.capelli@dstb.uniud.it

EYSTEIN ENOKSEN, Department of Sport and Biology, Norwegian University of Sport and Physical Education, P.B. 4014, U.S., 0806 Oslo, Norway. Telephone: (+47) 2326 2310 Fax: (+47) 2326 2451 E-mail: eysteine@nih.no

ALBERT GOLLHOFER, Department of Sport Science, Allmandring 28, 70569 Stuttgart. Telephone: (+49) 6853186 E-mail: Albert.Gollhofer@sport.uni-stuttgart.de

HENRIK B. LARSEN, Institute of Exercise and Sports Sciences, University of Copenhagen, Universitetsparken 13, 2100 Copenhagen Ø, Denmark. Telephone: (+45) 3675 5317 E-mail: hboegh@hotmail.com

T. D. NOAKES, Bioenergetics of Exercise Research Unit, University of Cape Town, Sports Science Institute of South Africa, Boundary Road Newlands, 7700, South Africa. Telephone: (021) 6867330 Fax: (021) 6867530 E-mail: TDNOAKES@SPORTS.UCT.AC.ZA

JAN SVEDENHAG, Department of Clinical Physiology, Karolinska Institute, S:t Göran Hospital, 112 81 Stockholm, Sweden. Telephone: (+46) 8 5870 1515 Fax: (+46) 8 5870 1928
E-mail: Jan.Svedenhag@stgoran.se

PIETRO E. DI PRAMPERO, Dipartimento di Scienze e Tecnologie Biomediche, School of Medicine, University of Udine, Via Gervasutta 48, 33100, Udine, Italy. Telephone: (+39) 432 520188 Fax: (+39) 432 600828

LEIF INGE TJELTA, Institute of Physical Education, Stavanger University College, P.O.Box 2557, Ullandhaug, 4091 Stavanger, Norway. Telephone: (+47) 5183 3523 Fax: (+47) 5183-3540
E-mail: leif.i.tjelta@lu.his.no

About the Editors

Jens Bangsbo is associate professor at the Institute of Exercise and Sport Sciences, University of Copenhagen, where he achieved his doctoral degree with the thesis „Physiology of Soccer – with a special reference to high intensity intermittent exercise". He has written more than one hundred original papers and reviews. He is the author of 12 books published in a number of different languages. He is a member of the Copenhagen Muscle Research Centre. He has received the „Biochemistry of Exercise" award. He is a member of the International Steering Group on Science and Football.

Henrik B. Larsen is a researcher at the August Krogh Institute, University of Copenhagen, where he has studied the physiology of running. He is author of many articles on different topics of sports physiology. He is a former 400 m runner and has represented Denmark on the junior national team. Furthermore, he is former national coach (1987-1995) for the Danish middle- and long distance runners. He is currently performing a number of scientific investigations attempting to reveal the reasons for the Kenyan superiority in middle- and long distance running.

About the Authors

Tim Noakes is professor of exercise and sports science at the University of Cape Town and the Sports Science Institute of South Africa. He has been an active runner for the past 30 years and completed more than 70 marathon or ultramarathon races including seven 90 km Comrades Marathon with a best time in 1973 of 06:49. He is author of the book "Lore of Running". His research interests include the nature of fatigue during exercise and factors that determine elite performance in sports like running, and in skill sports like cricket.

Jesper L. Andersen is a researcher at the Copenhagen Muscle Research Centre in the Department of Molecular Muscle Biology at the Copenhagen University Hospital in Copenhagen, Denmark. He did his PhD at the August Krogh Institute at the University of Copenhagen. He is the author of a number scientific articles published in international journals. Furthermore, he is former coach for the Danish National track and field team (sprinters).

Carlo Capelli is associate professor of human physiology at the School of Medicine of Udine, Italy. He is a medical doctor with a post doctorate education in Sports Medicine. He is the author of several papers dealing with the energy cost of human locomotion and has a particular interest in models utilised to predict best performances in sport.

Pietro Enrico di Prampero is professor of human physiology at the School of Medicine of Udine, Italy. He is author of several papers published on international journals of exercise and respiratory physiology and of one book on biomechanics and bioenergetics of human locomotion. He has been member of the Life Science Working Group and of the Microgravity Advisory Board of the European Space Agency. He is presently the editor-in-chief of the European Journal of Applied Physiology. He has particular interests in the exercise and respiratory physiology, in the physiology of the adaptation to microgravity in humans and in the bioenergetics applied to record performances in human locomotion.

Jan Svedenhag is associate professor in exercise physiology at the Karolinska Institute, Stockholm, Sweden. He is presently working at the Department of Clinical Physiology, S:t Görans Hospital, Stockholm. As a devoted long- distance runner (best marathon time 2:22) he became interested in the secrets of running. He has worked with the Swedish National Teams in middle- and long-distance running and triathlon as well as in cross-country skiing. Apart from exercise physiology, he has also particular interest in environmental physiology, such as the effect of altitude.

Albert Gollhofer is professor of biomechanics of the Department of Sport Science at the University of Stuttgart, Germany. He is president of the German Society of Biomechanics and serves as the head of the scientific committee of the European College of Sport Science. His engagements comprise several memberships in national and international editorial boards. The main research interest is related to neuro-muscular control mechanisms and their functional adaptations to training and exercise. In several research projects he investigates the biomechanics of joint stabilization of the ankle and knee joint complexes. He is author and co-author of numerous publications in this area.

Henrik B. Larsen is a researcher at the August Krogh Institute, University of Copenhagen, where he has studied the physiology of running. He is author of many articles on different topics of sports physiology. He is a former 400 m runner and has represented Denmark on the junior national team. Furthermore, he is former national coach (1987-1995) for the Danish middle- and long distance runners. He is currently performing a number of scientific investigations attempting to reveal the reasons for the Kenyan superiority in middle- and long distance running.

Leif Inge Tjelta is assistant professor in sport at Institute of Physical Education at Stavanger University College. He has been coaching distance runners for 20 years and have been National coach in Norway. He has competed international for Norway on 1500 m and was a distance runner of national standard until his late thirties. As member of the board in the Norwegian Association for Athletic Coaches, he has written many articles concerning distance running.

Eystein Enoksen is associate professor at the Norwegian University of Sport, Oslo, Norway. He is the leader of the department of track and field as well as the coaching education at the university. In addition, he has been consultant for the national association for coaches in track and field for ten years. He has 30 years of teaching and coaching experience in middle- and long distance training. He has written extensively in the fields of physical education, track and field, training theory/conditioning, recreation and health.

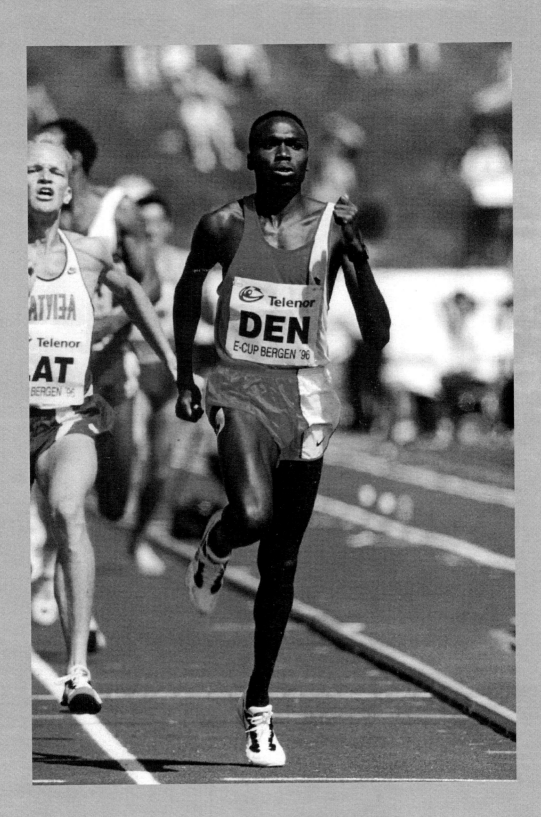

Physiological Capacity of the Elite Runner

Tim Noakes

Synopsis

The importance of conceptual models is that they indicate that different physiological systems may contribute to the success of elite athletes at different racing distances. In the past there has, perhaps, been an excessive focus on the exclusive role of cardiovascular function and oxygen transport in determining superior running performance. Rather this review suggests that multiple physiological systems likely contribute to superior running ability. The challenge for the coming generation of exercise physiologists is better to define the separate contributions of these different systems.

Introduction

The essential characteristics of the elite distance runner is the ability to sustain a high rate of energy expenditure (running speed) for unusually long. Indeed the most successful athletes are those who maintain this optimum rate of energy production for the entire duration of any race, seemingly without apparent fatigue. The range of these performances is also quite astonishing. Thus whereas the average human might be especially proud to run at 12 km•h^{-1} (5 min•km^{-1}) for 60 or so minutes, the best athletes in the world can run at better than 21 km•h^{-1} for 21 km, 20 km•h^{-1} for 42 km and 16.5 km•h^{-1} for 90 km, the latter lasting for close to 5½ hours. When it is appreciated that few humans, except trained athletes, can sustain a running speed of 16 km•h^{-1} for more than a few minutes, the unique ability of these elite athletes begins to become apparent.

In addition, any analysis of the world's best runners at distances from 5-42 km shows that all are also very fast over short distances of 800 m to the mile. For example, current 10000 m world record holder, Ethiopian Haile Gebrselassie has current (1999) fastest 800 and 1500 m times of 1:49.51 and 3:31.76 min, respectively. His closest rival at distances from 3000-10000 m, Kenyan Daniel Komen has already run the mile 1 second faster than one of the greatest milers of all time, former world record holder and double Olympic champion, Sebastian Coe. Yet when their respective best performances over 5000 m are compared, Komen's best current time is more than 80 seconds, or 10% faster than Coe's best at that distance (53).

It is rumoured that when Gebrselassie retires from competitive track running, he plans to be the first human to run the 42.2 km marathon in less than 2hrs, an improvement of more than 5 minutes on the current world record. Few knowledgeable in the sport would be prepared to bet against the possibility that either of these two athletes, unquestionably the most physiologically gifted runners of all time, will achieve this and other athletic records considered unattainable even quite recently.

In summary, an analysis of the physiological factors explaining superior running ability must explain both characteristics of the elite runners; the ability to run very fast in shorter distance races lasting from 90 seconds to 4 minutes, and the ability to run at a high percentage of that maximum speed for up to 2 or more hours. These two abilities may be caused by the same physiological variables, or they may be entirely different. We begin this analysis of these variables by evaluating the traditional physiological explanation for superior running ability before speculating on a more modern interpretation.

Maximum oxygen consumption as a predictor of running ability

A fundamental physiological principle is that the best predictor of a specific competitive performance is a laboratory or field test that closely mimics the duration of the actual competitive performance.

The original and still the most popular test to predict running ability is the measurement of maximum oxygen consumption ($\dot{V}O_2$-max). This test typically lasts less than 20 minutes for about the last quarter (2-5 minutes) of which the athlete is running under the duress similar to that experienced in competitions lasting a few minutes, such as races of 800-1500 m. The physiological logic for this test has been inherited from the studies of Hill et al. (30, 32) as interpreted by Taylor et al. (75).

It was originally assumed, since questioned by Noakes (48, 50, 51), that Hill and his colleagues had established that during progressive exercise to exhaustion, humans reached a "plateau" in oxygen consumption so that oxygen consumption failed to rise further despite further increases in running speed (Figure 1). As a result, continued running beyond the plateau was said to cause the muscles to contract anaerobically with production of lactic acid that ultimately prevented further muscle contraction, causing exhaustion and termination of exercise. Hence the assumption has been that a greater capacity to transport oxygen to the active muscles would delay the onset of anaerobic conditions in the active muscles, thereby allowing the athlete to continuing running for longer. As a result, a high capacity to transport oxygen would (a) be measured as a high $\dot{V}O_2$-max value; (b) would allow the athlete to achieve a high running speed during the $\dot{V}O_2$-max test, and (c) would be an excellent predictor of running ability at any running distance. There is now sufficient experience that the promise and pitfalls of the $\dot{V}O_2$-max test for predicting running ability are relatively well defined.

In the first place, it is established that those elite athletes who have the ability to achieve the fastest running speeds in competitions lasting more than 2 minutes have much higher $\dot{V}O_2$-max values, than do recreational athletes or untrained subjects (65). Given the linear relationship between oxygen consumption and running speed (Figure 1), it is to be expected that the best runners would reach higher running speeds and hence higher $\dot{V}O_2$-max values than less good athletes. Table 1 shows the range of $\dot{V}O_2$-max values recorded in some elite athletes.

One of the highest reported $\dot{V}O_2$-max value in a male runner is that of former 10000 m world record holder Dave Bedford (85 ml $O_2 \cdot kg^{-1} \cdot min^{-1}$) and in a female runner, 78 ml $O_2 \cdot kg^{-1} \cdot min^{-1}$ in Joan Benoit, winner of the inaugural 1984 Womens Olympic Marathon. The highest value yet reported in any athlete is a value of 93 ml $O_2 \cdot kg^{-1} \cdot min^{-1}$ in a

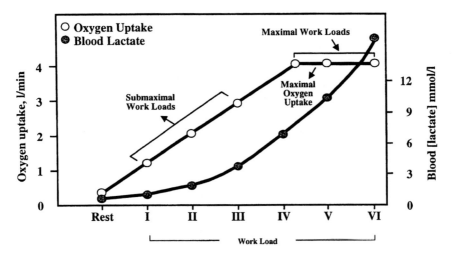

Figure 1. A popular graphic depicting how the original studies of Hill et al. were interpreted to indicate the development of a "plateau" that defined the maximum oxygen consumption ($\dot{V}O_2$-max).
Redrawn from 41.

Scandinavian cross-country skier. In contrast, $\dot{V}O_2$-max values measured in otherwise healthy young men are much lower, usually between 45 to 55 ml $O_2 \cdot kg^{-1} \cdot min^{-1}$, or about 40 percent lower than in elite athletes. As the $\dot{V}O_2$-max can be improved by up to a maximum of 20-25 percent even with intensive training, it is clear that the average healthy individual can train as much as he or she likes, yet will never achieve a $\dot{V}O_2$-max value anywhere near that of the elite athletes. Therefore, in as much as $\dot{V}O_2$-max is an (indirect) measure of potential for success in endurance activities, it is clear that hereditary factors must play an important role in determining those who will become champions.

But it is interesting that even among elite athletes with quite similar performances, $\dot{V}O_2$-max values may vary quite dramatically. For example, American runners Steve Prefontaine and Frank Shorter (Table 1), two athletes whose $\dot{V}O_2$-max values differed substantially (by 16 percent), had best mile times that differed by less than 8 seconds (3.4 percent) and best 3 mile (4.8 km) times that differed by even less (0.2 seconds). If $\dot{V}O_2$-max is the sole explanation for differences in running performance, then Prefontaine should have been much better at all running distances. Similarly, despite a substantially higher $\dot{V}O_2$-max value, Joan Benoit's marathon times were not faster than that of Derek

Clayton, who held the world marathon record despite a relatively poor $\dot{V}O_2$-max value of 69 ml $O_2 \cdot kg^{-1} \cdot min^{-1}$. These examples suggest that the $\dot{V}O_2$-max becomes a less good predictor of elite athletic performances as the distance of the event increases although this has not been scientifically evaluated. This too can be inferred from the comparison of the respective 5000 m performance of Sebastian Coe ($\dot{V}O_2$-max = 78 ml $O_2 \cdot kg^{-1} \cdot min^{-1}$) and Daniel Komen whose $\dot{V}O_2$-max has not been reported. It seem improbable that Komen's 10% faster time over 5000 m but similar 1500 m time as Coe could be due to a substantially higher $\dot{V}O_2$-max than that of Coe.

The alternate paradox is that some athletes with quite similar $\dot{V}O_2$-max values have quite different running performances. Compare, for example, the performances of the American, Alberto Salazar, the Norwegian, Grete Waitz and the Briton, Cavin Woodward, whose best marathon times of 2:08:13; 2:25:29 and 2:19:50 hr:min:s, respectively, were greatly different despite similar $\dot{V}O_2$-max values (Table 1).

In summary, the $\dot{V}O_2$-max test, long considered the ultimate predictor of running performance has been shown to have limitations. First, the test is an excellent predictor of performance in groups of

Table 1. Maximum oxygen consumption ($\dot{V}O_2$-max) and performance values of some elite runners

Athlete	Country	Major performance	$\dot{V}O_2$-max (ml•kg⁻¹•min⁻¹)
David Bedford	UK	10000 m WR (1973)	85
Steve Prefontaine	USA	1 mile 03:54.6	84
Craig Virgin	USA	2:10:26 Marathon	81
Joan Benoit	USA	1984 Olympic Marathon gold medal	78
Sebastian Coe	UK	1980 and 1984 1500 m Olympic Gold medals	78
Alberto Salazar	USA	Marathon WR (1981)	76
Cavin Woodward	UK	100 km WR (1976)	74
Grete Waitz	Norway	Marathon WR (1980)	73
Frank Shorter	USA	1972 Olympic Marathon gold medal	71
Derek Clayton	Australia	Marathon WR (1969)	69

WR = World Record

23

athletes of quite different abilities including the very good and the very bad. When this approach is used, the results are as expected. The slow athletes have low $\dot{V}O_2$-max values, the fast runners much higher $\dot{V}O_2$-max values (2, 13, 14, 17, 23, 24, 39, 42, 77).

However, when groups of athletes with very similar running performances are studied, for example, the athletes listed in Table 1, then, it is found that the $\dot{V}O_2$-max becomes a far less sensitive predictor of performance (9, 10, 11, 12, 54, 59, 65, 69).

Furthermore, the predictive ability of the $\dot{V}O_2$-max test becomes less the longer the duration of the competitive event. This however should not be surprising. For the reason that the $\dot{V}O_2$-max test is of relatively short duration and, in essence, involves running at close to maximum speed for a few minutes, similar to the demands of racing 800-2000 m. According to the concept of specificity of testing, it would be likely that this test would predict performance more accurately in short-duration events of high intensity than it would during more prolonged exercise when factors other than the maximum capacity to transport oxygen, might determine performance. These factors could relate to skeletal muscle or perhaps even central (brain) function (53).

Why the $\dot{V}O_2$-max test is not a flawless predictor of running ability

Running economy and peak treadmill running speed

The first reason why the $\dot{V}O_2$-max test alone is a relatively less good predictor of running performance is because athletes differ (i) in their rate of oxygen consumption ($\dot{V}O_2$) at any running speed and (ii) in the peak running speed they reach during the maximal treadmill test. David Dill and his colleagues (20) and later David Costill's group (12, 15) were probably the first scientists to suggest that there may be differences in the amount of oxygen different athletes actually require when running at the same speeds. These individual differences in running economy and in peak treadmill running velocity could be the factors explaining different running performance in athletes with similar $\dot{V}O_2$-max values or conversely similar running performance in athletes with very dissimilar $\dot{V}O_2$-max values (48). Figure 2 which compares the $\dot{V}O_2$ at

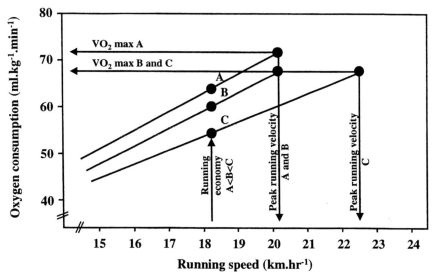

Figure 2. Comparison of running economy, peak treadmill running speed and $V O_2$-max in three theoretical runners (A, B and C) who differ in their running economy and peak treadmill running velocity, defined as the peak treadmill velocity achieved during the progressive exercise test for measurement of $V O_2$-max.

Note that the least economical runner A achieves the same peak treadmill velocity as runner B but has the highest $V O_2$-max; the more economical runner B achieves the same peak treadmill velocity and hence a lower $V O_2$-max than runner A; whereas the most economical runner C achieves the highest peak treadmill velocity with a $V O_2$-max only equal to that of runner B and lower than that of runner A.

submaximal running speeds (running economy) and the maximal running velocity, as well as the $\dot{V}O_2$-max in 3 idealised runners A, B and C, explains this phenomenon.

The first difference between the three runners is their oxygen consumption at any submaximal running speed. Hence, as shown in Figure 2, runner C is the most economical runner as his $\dot{V}O_2$ at 18 km•h^{-1} is about 55 ml O_2•kg^{-1}•min^{-1} whereas B and A are less economical with $\dot{V}O_2$'s of about 60 ml O_2•kg^{-1}•min^{-1} and 65 ml O_2•kg^{-1}•min^{-1} respectively. The first result is that when runners A and B reach their peak treadmill running speeds at 20 km•h^{-1}, the least economical runner, runner A, has a higher $\dot{V}O_2$-max value than does runner B. Yet the most economical runner, runner C, reaches a higher peak treadmill running velocity than both runners A and B, yet his $\dot{V}O_2$-max is equal to that of B but lower than that of A. But which of these runners would likely run the fastest in races of 3-21 km?

25

In general, it has been shown that the best athletes are usually the most economical (48) corresponding to runner C in Figure 2. This finding has been most clearly shown by Conley and Krahenbuhl (10), who studied a group of 12 runners whose best 10 km times were closely bunched between 30:31 and 33:33 min. They found that the runners' $\dot{V}O_2$-max values, which ranged from 67 to 78 ml $O_2 \cdot kg^{-1} \cdot min^{-1}$, could not be used to predict their 10 km times. For example, the second-fastest runner had the second-lowest $\dot{V}O_2$-max value. However, there was an excellent correlation between the $\dot{V}O_2$ of each runner at each of three submaximal running speeds (14.5, 16.1 and 17.7 $km \cdot h^{-1}$) and their best time for the 10 km race. Thus the runners who used the least oxygen at each of these running speeds and were therefore the most economical, had the fastest 10 km running times.

The authors concluded that a high $\dot{V}O_2$-max (above 67 ml $O_2 \cdot kg^{-1} \cdot min^{-1}$) helped each athlete gain membership of this elite performance group, but within this select group, running economy and not $\dot{V}O_2$-max was the factor controlling success in the 10 km race.

But I would interpret these data somewhat differently. For according to Figure 2, athletes with different running economies and similar $\dot{V}O_2$-max values must differ in the peak treadmill speed that they achieve during the $\dot{V}O_2$-max test (compare runners B and C). Or else their $\dot{V}O_2$-max values must be different (compare runners A and B). Thus the crucial, but unreported physiological data, necessary for a full analysis of the study of Conley and Krahenbuhl (10), was the peak treadmill running velocities achieved by their subjects during the maximal exercise test. We have defined this as the peak running velocity achieved during the progressive exercise test used for the measurement of the $\dot{V}O_2$-max (48, 54).

For there are now a number of studies showing that the peak treadmill running velocity is at least as good as any other variable and substantially superior to the $\dot{V}O_2$-max, for predicting running performance at a range of distances (4, 28, 34, 36, 37, 38, 43, 54, 57, 69, 70, 78).

Thus, according to these predictions, Runner C in Figure 2 would be the fastest runner at any distance despite having a lower $\dot{V}O_2$-max value than Runner A. The low $\dot{V}O_2$-max is a reflection of a superior running economy; his superior performance is related to his ability to achieve the highest peak treadmill running speed. The runner in Table 1 who most closely fits this description would be Derek Clayton, who is known to have been one of the most economical runners yet studied, who had a relatively low $\dot{V}O_2$-max (Table 1) but who nevertheless held the world record for the 42 km standard marathon.

In contrast, runner A performs less well than his high $\dot{V}O_2$-max would predict because he is the least economical of the three runners and only reaches the same peak treadmill speed as does runner B, despite a higher $\dot{V}O_2$-max. Hence his performances would likely be similar to those of runner B and would be inferior to that of runner C, whose $\dot{V}O_2$-max value is lower.

The runners in Table 1 who would best fit the characteristics of runner A are Americans Craig Virgin and Joan Benoit and Norwegian Grete Waitz, all of whose performances appear less good than their high $\dot{V}O_2$-max values would predict.

Differences in fatigue resistance

One of the most interesting recent phenomena in athletics has been the rise of East African, especially Kenyan, runners to a position of unmatched dominance especially in the 3000 m steeplechase and the 12 km cross country events (52). Currently Kenyans win between 40 and 50% of all medals in international competitions from 800 m to the marathon. No international sport has ever been dominated to such an extent by athletes from one country (1).

Two studies of Kenyan runners (66, 67, 68) have so far failed to provide a definitive physiological answer for their manifest superiority as distance runners. The overriding conclusion was that the Kenyans' $\dot{V}O_2$-max values were not inordinately high. In the words of the senior author, Professor Bengt Saltin: "A comparison of some data on some of the very best runners in Kenya during the last decades and world class runners in Scandinavia does not reveal much that was not already known or could be anticipated" (68).

The only other study of elite (South) African distance runners is that of Coetzer et al. (9). That study reported physiological data in one of the best group of distance runners yet evaluated anywhere in the world. The physiological characteristics of a group of South African distance runners were compared to those of South African middle distance runners. Running performances of both groups were similar at race distances up to 3 km. But the performances of the distance runners became significantly better at the longer distances. Table 2 lists the important findings of that study.

The African distance runners were lighter and smaller, as also reported by Saltin (68), with a slightly lower proportion of Type I muscle fibres. But the key finding was that the distance runners were able to run substantially faster at all distances beyond 5 km despite $\dot{V}O_2$-max values that were the same as those of the middle distance runners. Hence the measurement of $\dot{V}O_2$-max alone failed to explain the superior endurance capacity of the (South) African distance runners in that study and also in the studies of Saltin and colleagues (66, 67).

Rather, the important difference was that the long distance runners were able to sustain a substantially higher proportion of their $\dot{V}O_2$-max when racing. This is shown graphically in Figure 3, which compares the % $\dot{V}O_2$-max sustained by the long distance and middle distance runners at different racing distances. At distances beyond 5 km, the distance runners sustained a significantly higher % $\dot{V}O_2$-max than did the middle distance runners and the difference increased with increasing racing distance. Thus the crucial finding was that the superior performance of the distance runners with increasing running distance

Table 2. Physiological comparison of elite South African long distance and middle distance runners

	Middle distance	Long distance
Maximal aerobic power ($ml \cdot kg^{-1} \cdot min^{-1}$)	72	71
Muscle fibre composition (% Type I)	63	53*
Height (cm)	181	169*
Weight (kg)	70	56*
Fatigue resistance (% $\dot{V}O_{2max}$ for 21 km)	82	89*

*Data from 9.   *p <0.05.*

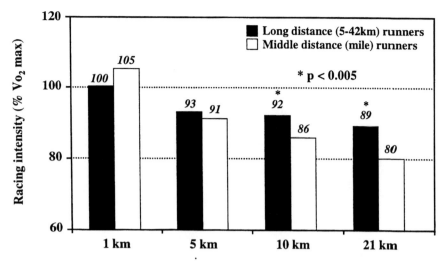

Figure 3. The exercise intensity (% $\dot{V}O_{2max}$) sustained by two groups of elite South African athletes differing in the race distances at which they specialize. Note that the long distance runners sustain a significantly higher running intensity at all race distances beyond 10 km.

was explained by their superior fatigue resistance and was not due to a higher maximal aerobic power ($\dot{V}O_2$-max) than the middle-distance runners (Table 2). Other studies have also found that (South) African distance runners have superior fatigue resistance when compared to sub-elite Caucasian runners of similar abilities (7, 76).

Hence, the important finding of that study was that the $\dot{V}O_2$-max may be unable to discriminate between good and superior performance in events lasting more than a few minutes and which constitute the bulk of sporting events. The failure stems from the inability of this model to measure or predict fatigue resistance during prolonged sub-maximal exercise on the basis of physiological variables and performance measured during a single bout of progressive, maximal exercise to exhaustion in a test that lasts only a few minutes.

Further support for this explanation can be surmised from other information in Figure 3, which shows that these athletes run at 100% or greater of their $\dot{V}O_2$ max in race distances of 1-2 km. Yet it is not at those distances that the Kenyans are anymore dominant than they are at the longer racing distances. If the Kenyans' success was due to their unusually high $\dot{V}O_2$-max values, one would expect their athletes to be more dominant at 800 metres to the mile than at other distances. This is not the case (52).

In summary, the concept that endurance athletes differ in their fatigue resistance is not new; a number of studies have shown that athletes differ in the exercise intensity expresses as a $\%\dot{V}O_2$-max, that each can sustain during more prolonged exercise (13, 17) and that this variable also predicts endurance performance.

What has perhaps not always been appreciated is that physiological factors determining the $\dot{V}O_2$-max and the $\%\dot{V}O_2$-max that can be sustained during prolonged exercise might be quite different so that a high $\dot{V}O_2$-max value does not guarantee the capacity to sustain a high $\dot{V}O_2$-max during more prolonged exercise, and vice versa.

Hence another possible explanation for the differences in running performance of athletes with different or similar $\dot{V}O_2$-max values (Table 1) is likely to be differences in the $\%\dot{V}O_2$-max that each can sustain during prolonged exercise. Some possible explanations for this are described subsequently.

Concerns with the $\dot{V}O_2$-max model for predicting athletic ability

A final reason why the $\dot{V}O_2$-max may be a relatively poor predictor of athletic ability in runners with similar abilities could possibly be because performance may not actually be determined by the rate of oxygen delivery to the active muscles and the prevention of anaerobic skeletal muscle metabolism, as is usually assumed. The arguments against this theory have been detailed (48; 50, 51, 53) and only the salient points will be reviewed here.

The theoretical basis for the model which uses the $\dot{V}O_2$-max to predict running performance, holds that the "plateau" in oxygen consumption during the $\dot{V}O_2$-max test occurs when the heart is unable to increase the cardiac output. As a result, blood flow to the exercising muscles reaches a maximum value. Hence any further increase in work output by the exercising muscles can only be achieved by an increase in anaerobic metabolism with the production of lactate and hydrogen ions (H^+). Accumulation of lactate and H^+ are then thought to inhibit muscular contraction causing the termination of exercise.

Perhaps the major but overlooked limitation of this model is that, if the pumping capacity of the heart does indeed limit oxygen utilization by the exercising skeletal muscle, then the heart itself will be the first organ affected by any postulated oxygen deficiency (51, 53). This was first recognized by Hill and his colleagues as early as 1924 (32) yet was lost to posterity until recently re-discovered (51, 53).

For the interpretation of Hill and his colleagues was unequivocal: "Certain it is that the capacity of the body for muscular exercise depends largely, if not mainly, on the capacity and output of the heart. It would obviously be very dangerous for the organ to be able, as the skeletal muscle is able, to exhaust itself very completely and rapidly, to take exercise far in excess of it capacity for recovery. ...When the oxygen supply becomes inadequate, it is probable that the heart rapidly begins to diminish its output, so avoiding exhaustion..." (32).

The point identified by Hill and his colleagues and since seems to be overlooked by subsequent generations of exercise physiologists, is that the heart is also a muscle, dependant for its function on an adequate blood and oxygen supply. But, unlike skeletal muscle, the heart is dependent for its blood supply on its own pumping capacity. Hence any intervention that reduces the pumping capacity of the heart, or demands the heart somehow to sustain an increased work output by the exercising muscles without any increase in cardiac output and coronary flow (as theoretically occurs when the "plateau phenomenon" develops), must imperil the heart's own blood supply. Any reduction in coronary blood flow will consequently reduce the heart's pumping capacity, thereby inducing a vicious cycle of progressive and irreversible myocardial ischaemia. It would seem logical that human design should include controls to protect the heart from ever entering this vicious circle.

Hence if (skeletal) muscle function fails when its oxygen demand exceeds supply then, for logical consistency, the inability of the pumping capacity of the heart to increase the cardiac output at the supposed $\dot{V}O_2$-max plateau, must also result from an inadequate (myocardial) oxygen supply caused by a plateau in coronary flow. This limiting coronary blood flow induces myocardial "fatigue", causing the plateau in cardiac output and hence in the $\dot{V}O_2$-max leading, finally, to skeletal muscle anaerobiosis. Thus, by this logic, the coronary blood flow must be the first physiological function to show a "plateau phenomenon" during progressive exercise to exhaustion. All subsequent physiological "plateaus" must result from this limiting coronary flow.

31

Perhaps the reluctance of modern physiologists to embrace these concepts stems from the current appreciation that progressive myocardial ischaemia does not occur during maximal exercise in healthy athletes (60), even though there is good evidence that it is a limiting cardiac output that probably determines the VO_2-max (64). Thus one postulate might be that even if cardiac output limits maximal exercise as seems likely, termination of exercise must occur before the heart actually reaches that maximum and hence well before skeletal muscle anaerobiosis can develop. Hence for 75 years, exercise physiologists may have focused on the incorrect organ as the site of any potential anaerobiosis that may develop during maximal exercise (32).

In summary, there may be a fundamental physiological flaw in the model which holds that anaerobic metabolism occurs in skeletal muscle during maximal exercise when the oxygen demands of the muscles exceed the heart's maximum capacity to match that demand. Not least because the model predicts that a "plateau" in cardiac output must develop before skeletal muscle anaerobiosis can begin to occur. But any "plateau" in cardiac output requires that myocardial ischaemia be present either to cause that plateau, according to the theory that anaerobiosis limits muscle function, or as a result of it, as the cardiac output determines both coronary and skeletal muscle blood flow. As myocardial ischaemia has never been shown to develop during maximal exercise in healthy humans, so would it seem unlikely that skeletal muscle anaerobiosis can develop during progressive exercise to exhaustion. Indeed no study has yet conclusively shown convincing biochemical or other evidence for skeletal muscle anaerobiosis during maximum exercise (27, 62). Rather skeletal muscle oxygenation does not appear to alter in the transition from rest to maximum exercise (33, 62), a finding that severely taxes any theory that skeletal muscle anaerobiosis develops during exercise or that the products of anaerobic metabolism limit maximum exercise. Rather I have argued that there may be a neural (brain) mechanism that terminates exercise before the onset of either skeletal muscle or myocardial anaerobiosis.

Whilst this mechanism is designed to protect the heart from myocardial ischaemia, only indirectly does it determine the actual peak work rate achieved during maximal exercise (Figure 4). For the actual peak work rate achieved will depend on the "quality" of the skeletal and cardiac muscle. Superior myocardial contractility and efficiency of oxygen use would increase the maximum cardiac output achieved

Physiological factors that may limit maximal exercise performance.

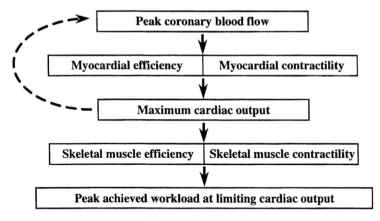

Figure 4. Postulated physiological factors that may limit maximal exercise performance.

Note that this model predicts that a peak coronary blood flow may limit exercise by activating a neural (brain) reflex which prevents any further increase in skeletal muscle recruitment in the active muscles. The peak running velocity (Figure 2) at that maximal coronary blood flow will, in turn, be determined by the efficiency and contractility of both the heart and the active skeletal muscles.

at any maximum (limiting) coronary flow. Similarly at any maximum skeletal muscle blood flow, superior contractility and efficiency of skeletal muscle contraction would increase the peak work rate or running velocity (Figure 2) achieved at that maximum cardiac output.

Thus this analysis of what I have termed the traditional Cardiovascular/Anaerobic Model of Exercise Physiology and Athletic Performance (53) leads to the alternate hypothesis that superior fatigue resistance, determined perhaps by the central nervous system, or by skeletal muscle contractile function, might explain superior performance in events lasting more than a few minutes. This superior fatigue resistance cannot be predicted by the Cardiovascular/Anaerobic Model which uses exercise tests of short duration and in which the fatigue resistance component of endurance performance is not measured. By extension, it would seem that fatigue resistance is not causally determined by the magnitude of the athlete's cardiovascular capacity, although maximum exercise capacity in events of 2-15 minutes is very likely to be influenced predominantly by cardiovascular function and, especially, the peak

33

coronary blood flow (Figure 4). There is also no logical reason to believe that fatigue resistance during submaximal exercise is determined by either the presence or absence of skeletal muscle anaerobiosis (62).

Accordingly differences in endurance capacity in events lasting more than about 15 minutes are unlikely to be determined solely by differences in cardiovascular function. With the exception that high rates of maximum coronary blood flow would likely be crucial to sustain the very high maximal cardiac outputs and hence high $\dot{V}O_2$-max values achieved during exercise lasting less than 10-15 minutes.

Thus, this analysis suggests that the very best athletes have very high exercise capacities not primarily because they are able to increase oxygen supply to their exercising muscles but because of a high capacity to increase blood flow to their hearts. In addition, superior efficiency and contractility of their hearts and skeletal muscles would ensure that very high running speeds are achieved at that limiting rate of blood flow to the heart.

For further consideration regarding this hypothesis please see Bassett & Howley (2a) and Bergh et al. (2b).

Models to evaluate differences in fatigue resistance between athletes

Since it has been assumed for the past 75 years that differences in running ability must result solely from differences in their maximum ability to transport and utilise oxygen, so the possibility that other factors may influence performance have been somewhat ignored. Currently, there are at least three other possible explanations for superior exercise capacity and fatigue resistance during more prolonged exercise.

The energy depletion model to explain superior performance in marathon and ultramarathon running events

There is good evidence that fatigue during prolonged exercise develops coincidentally with the achievement of very low liver and muscle glycogen concentrations, the former causing a low blood glucose concentration (hypoglycaemia) (3, 16). Ingestion of carbohydrate during exercise enhances performance, perhaps by delaying the onset of hypo-glycaemia (53).

Thus one possibility is that superior fatigue resistance in events lasting more than 90-120 minutes and in which either liver or muscle glycogen depletion might cause fatigue, could result from a greater capacity of some athletes either (i) to store more muscle and liver glycogen before exercise, or (ii) to produce glucose more readily in the liver during exercise, or (iii) to slow the rate of muscle or liver glycogen use during exercise. There is little scientific evidence that any or all of these adaptations can specifically explain the superior performances of elite athletes and any conclusions in this regard are currently speculative.

But during very prolonged competitive exercise lasting more than 6 hours, depletion of body carbohydrate stores must occur regardless of any metabolic adaptations that may have occurred in the athlete's carbohydrate metabolism.

For example, it is currently difficult to explain performance in ultra-endurance events, especially the final 42 km running leg of 226 km ironman triathlon events according to a model which holds that exercise of moderately-high intensity ($> 65\%$ $\dot{V}O_2$-max) is not possible once there is marked muscle glycogen depletion. After cycling at 40 km•h^{-1} for 4.5 h, the elite triathletes, the best of whom are also exceptional runners, would be expected to have near total muscle glycogen depletion according to data from laboratory studies (6, 8). The studies of Rauch et al. (61) and O'Brien et al. (56) suggest that total carbohydrate oxidation during very prolonged exercise of up to 6 hrs duration exceeds the estimated carbohydrate stores in liver and active muscle by up to 100%. Yet the best performers in that event are still able to run at close to 16 km•h^{-1} for a further 160 minutes. This probably represents an exercise intensity of $> 66\%$ $\dot{V}O_2$-max. Either these calcu-lations are incorrect, or other sources of carbohydrate, in addition to those in the active muscles and liver, must contribute to fuel oxidation in events lasting more than 4-6 hours.

However the equally plausible alternate theory postulates that superior endurance capacity may be determined by the exact opposite; by a superior capacity to oxidise fat and hence maintain a lower respi-ratory quotient (RQ) during prolonged exercise. The latter possibility is supported by at least some evidence. In the studies of Bosch et.al. (8), those athletes unable to complete 3 hours of exercise at 70% VO_2-max after carbohydrate-loading had significantly higher RQ during exercise and were therefore characterised by an inability to sustain high rates of fat oxidation during prolonged exercise. Indeed simulated metabolic balance studies for the 226 km Hawaiian Ironman triathlon suggest it to be very likely that the capacity to oxidise fat at high rates will influence running speed late in events lasting more than 4-6 hours when muscle glycogen stores are likely to be depleted (53).

For example, our calculations suggest that an athlete cycling at 40 km•h^{-1} for 4.5 hours during the Ironman Triathlon would exercise at a $\dot{V}O_2$ of 57 ml•kg^{-1}•min^{-1}. To maintain this speed for 4.5 hrs of cycling, would require an elite male Ironman triathlete to oxidise about 700 g of carbohydrate and 175 g of fat. This compares to predicted whole body carbohydrate and fat stores of 520 g and 5000 g respectively. Hence this model predicts that, at the end of the cycle leg, an elite athlete would have depleted his body carbohydrate stores, yet must still run 42.2 km at close to 16 km•h^{-1}, if he wishes to be successful.

Our other laboratory data suggest that after 4.5 hrs of such exercise, the carbohydrate contribution to whole body energy metabolism would comprise a blood glucose oxidation rate of 1.2 g•min^{-1} (21 kJ•min^{-1}) and a lactate oxidation rate of 0.6 g•min^{-1} (10.5 kJ•min^{-1}). Together with the average maximum rate of fat oxidation that we have measured after 6 hours of laboratory cycling (0.76 g•min^{-1}; 28 kJ•min^{-1}), this provides a total rate of energy production of 59.5 kJ•min^{-1}. This would provide energy at a rate sufficient to sustain a running speed of approximately 12 km•h^{-1}, sufficient to complete the 42 km marathon leg of the Ironman Triathlon in 3 hr 30 mins. To equal the best marathon time yet run in that race, the athlete would be required to oxidize fat at a rate of 1.15 g•min^{-1}. This rate is approximately 50% faster than we have measured in cyclists in our laboratory.

Accordingly if this model of performance in very prolonged exercise is correct, then the difference between running the final 42 km marathon leg of an ironman triathlon in 2 hr 40 min versus 3 hr 30 min may simply be a 51% (0.4 g•min^{-1}) greater capacity to oxidize fat when body carbohydrate and, especially, muscle glycogen stores are depleted. By extension, the same adaptation could explain the superior running ability of ultramarathon racers.

The biomechanical model to explain superior running ability in middle to long distance running events

There is growing interest in the role of muscles as elastic energy return systems which function both as springs and torque producers during exercise (57, 63). Central to this model is the prediction that the greater the muscle's capacity to act as a spring, the less torque it must produce and hence the more efficient it is. The more efficient, more elastic muscle will enhance exercise performance, especially in weight-bearing activities like running, by slowing (i) the rate of accumulation of those metabolites that may cause fatigue during exercise and (ii) the rate of rise of body temperature thereby slowing the rate at which the core body temperature rises during exercise and (iii) by reducing the extent of muscle damage induced by repetitive eccentric muscle contraction especially of the quadriceps and calf muscles.

This new information underscores another important logical weakness of the Cardiovascular/Anaerobic Model for explaining enhanced endurance performance. For that model predicts that superior performance during prolonged exercise results from an increased oxygen delivery to muscle and an increased rate of energy and hence heat production. Thus according to that model, the price of running faster is that more heat must be produced. But a higher rate of heat production would induce fatigue prematurely due to excessive heat accumulation, according to the findings of Nielsen and her colleagues (26, 45, 46, 47). A more logical biological adaptation would be to reduce the rate of oxygen consumption and hence the rate of heat production by increasing the athlete's efficiency (economy) of movement. We have already noted that the best distance runners are usually those who are the most economical (Figure 2) so that this theory has some theoretical support.

Indeed, if the rate of heat accumulation limits exercise performance under specific conditions, then factors that slow the rate at which heat accumulates when running fast should enhance performance. Two such factors are small size (19) and superior running economy. A smaller size reduces the amount of heat produced when running at any speed. When environmental conditions limit the capacity for heat loss, smaller runners will be favoured (19). Indeed it is of interest that the average height and mass of the winners of the Boston (USA) marathon has not changed over the past 100 years despite an average increase in height of 1 cm per decade in Americans during the same time (55).

Further evidence supporting this argument that heat accumulation is a factor limiting endurance performance, is the finding that race times in both the marathon (49) and the longer distance track races including the 3000 m steeplechase and the 10000 m (40) deteriorate as the environmental heat load increases. Thus there is an inverse relationship between the environmental heat load, measured as the Wet Bulb Globe Temperature Index, and the reduction in race performance. It is well established that the ability to exercise in the laboratory is dependent on the environmental heat load (25). Furthermore, precooling, so that athletes begin exercise with lower body temperatures, enhances exercise performance (5).

Therefore, according to this model, the more economical the athlete, the faster he or she will be able to run before reaching a limiting body temperature. A number of studies indicate that the best endurance athletes are also frequently the most economical (49). Indeed most training studies show that improvements in running economy are perhaps the most likely response to training especially in those who are already well-trained (71). This adaptation allows the athlete to run faster at the same oxygen consumption; thus he or she completes a given distance more rapidly for the same average rate of heat accumulation but a reduced overall heat expenditure. This would be advantageous under conditions in which the heat load on the athlete increases, for example in marathon or longer races that continue into the mid- or late morning heat.

In contrast, a high maximum aerobic capacity, often a marker of poor running economy (49), would likely cause more rapid rates of heat accumulation and hence the more rapid onset of fatigue during prolonged exercise. This finding alone could explain why the best marathon runners usually have $\dot{V}O_2$-max values in the range of 69-74 $ml \cdot O_2 \cdot kg^{-1} \cdot min^{-1}$. Less economical runners with higher $\dot{V}O_2$-max values (48) have not necessarily been more successful (49). Figure 2 again offers the visual explanation for this phenomenon.

Thus this model predicts that success in endurance events is not likely to result from training that makes the athlete ever more powerful with a larger muscle mass and greater $\dot{V}O_2$-max. A more likely adaptation would be to reduce the athlete's size and increase his or her running efficiency. That runners believe they run better when lighter, is well known.

Another African analogy for this prediction is provided by the physiological strategy that the cheetah has evolved to survive as a successful predator. The cheetah, whose chase is terminated by an elevated rectal temperature after running at up to 100 km•h^{-1} for less than a minute (74), succeeds because of the animal's small size and probably a high degree of running economy (due to elasticity provided by the flexible spine). Thus laboratory experiments showed that when the cheetah's rectal temperature reached between 40.5 to 41°C, the cheetahs refused to run. They would simply turn over with their feet in the air and slide on the tread(mill) surface (74). This is analogous to humans who terminate exercise when a certain rectal temperature is achieved (26, 47).

The small size of the cheetah and its likely high running economy slows its rate of heat accumulation just sufficiently for it to outrun the smaller gazelles (~ 25 kg) on which it preys and whose escape is also restrained by a rising body temperature (73). Thus the chase between the gazelle and the cheetah is probably decided by which individual animal accumulates heat more slowly during the chase. In contrast, the heavier, more muscular lion has evolved a different, co-operative, hunting strategy, targeting larger but slower mammals.

Perhaps the point is that smallness and greater running economy would seem to be a technique used to increase endurance capacity in one animal, the cheetah. Logic suggests that this technique may also be applicable to elite human athletes.

A second component of the biomechanical models stems from the accumulating evidence that repeated high velocity, short duration eccentric muscle contractions, as occur during running, induce a specific form of fatigue that develops during running races and is measurable for at least 7 days after a marathon race (35, 44).

Characteristics of this fatigue are a failure of the contractile capacity of the exercised muscles with a reduced tolerance to muscle stretch and a delayed transfer from muscle stretch to muscle shortening in the stretch/shortening cycle. As a result, the durations of both the braking and push off phases in the running stride are increased, leading to mechanical changes in the stride with landing occurring on a more extended leg but with greater subsequent knee flexion at the onset of weight bearing.

As these abnormalities persists for many days after the race, they cannot be explained by acute changes in oxygen or substrate delivery to the muscles, or by the elevated body temperature during exercise, as required by the other models of fatigue presented here. Rather Komi and Nicol (35) conclude that: "Stretch shortening fatigue results usually in a reversible muscle damage process and has considerable influence on muscle mechanics, joint and muscle stiffness as well as on reflex intervention." Thus any evaluation of fatigue resistance, especially in weight-bearing activities like running, needs to consider this specific form of stretch/shortening cycle fatigue.

To return to the African analogy, empirical observation of the running stride and the anatomical structure of the lower limb of Kenyan runners suggests, at least to this author, that an evaluation of the elastic elements of the legs of elite Kenyan runners and their resistance to stretch/shortening cycle fatigue would likely be very rewarding.

For example, it appears that African athletes generally train harder than do Caucasian runners (9, 72). Especially the training volumes and intensities of the Kenyan runners (72) are unmatched by other athletes. But to achieve such training volumes, there must be superior resistance to the stretch/shortening cycle damage proposed by Komi and Nicol (35), both in training and in marathon racing.

Hence another possibility is that the more elastic muscles of elite distance runners are better able to resist eccentrically-induced damage in training. This may allow more intensive daily training and hence superior adaptations to training. That same superiority would also enhance performance during competitive racing by delaying the onset of this stretch/shortening cycle fatigue that is an inevitable consequence of repeated eccentric muscle contractions.

In summary, the biomechanical model predicts that superior performance especially in a weight-bearing activity like running, may be influenced by the capacity of the muscles to act as elastic energy-return systems. Changes in the efficiency and durability of this process would (i) enhance movement economy and reduce the rate of heat production during exercise, thereby enhancing exercise capacity by slowing the rate at which the body temperature rises when environmental conditions are severe; (ii) enhance the quality of training by allowing more rapid recovery from stretch/shortening cycle fatigue so that more frequent bouts of intensive training can be undertaken and (iii) enhance fatigue resistance during competition by increasing resistance to that form of muscle damage that develops during repeated cycles of stretch/shortening contractions.

The psychological/motivational model to explain superior running ability

This model holds that the ability to sustain exercise performance results from a conscious effort so that central (brain) fatigue (18) may contribute to the fatigue experienced during prolonged exercise. This interpretation conflicts with the other models which hold that exercise performance is regulated at a subconscious level and that such controls exist, in part, to prevent conscious override that might damage the human.

It would seem that exercise performance must include at least some component that can be influenced by conscious effort. The dichotomy of physiology and psychology has generally prevented adequate laboratory evaluation of this model. Any studies showing an ergogenic effect of any placebo intervention on exercise performance would prove that this model contributes, in part, to athletic performance. This is an area requiring a heightened research effort. For example, some suggest that the more demanding lifestyle of the Kenyan youth, including initiation rites and circumcision without anaesthesia, induce a different approach to pain than is perhaps present in populations without such rituals.

Conclusion

This chapter has reviewed some of the models currently promoted to predict the physiological variables that determine superior athletic ability. It has extended that analysis beyond a simple analysis of oxygen transport capacity. The insights offered by that broader view suggests that the following are likely to contribute to the superior exercise capacity of elite runners.

Cardiovascular system

Relevant physiological adaptations would be those that result in an increased $\dot{V}O_2$-max and skeletal muscle blood flow during both maximal exercise and increased muscle blood flow during prolonged submaximal exercise.

41

According to the model I have presented here, a plateau in coronary flow would appear to be the factor that would ultimately limit the cardiac output and hence the $\dot{V}O_2$-max. Thus an essential physiological attribute of the elite runner would be a very large maximal coronary flow. As the peak coronary blood flow is likely related to the mass of the heart, this would also explain why the hearts of the elite athletes are likely to be large and, because of the greater peak coronary blood flow rates, also capable of very high cardiac outputs.

However, even if elite athletes have a greater coronary flow, the actual peak work rate or peak $\dot{V}O_2$-max that each achieves will depend on the contractile state of the myocardium and the efficiency with which the heart is able to convert that maximum coronary flow into a peak cardiac output. Similarly the actual maximum work rate or running velocity achieved at the $\dot{V}O_2$-max, will equally depend on the economy and contractility of the skeletal muscles (Figure 4).

Thus the very best athletes would not only have very high rates of coronary flow but also superior efficiency and contractility of both the heart and skeletal muscles. Indeed there is a need better to understand the contractile characteristics of the skeletal muscles of superior athletes (22). Too often it has been assumed that skeletal muscle contractility is the same in all humans including athletes, an unlikely assumption (21, 22).

Energy depletion model

A reduced rate of carbohydrate utilization during prolonged exercise would enhance performance by delaying the onset of whole body carbohydrate depletion. This model predicts why an increased capacity to burn fat during prolonged exercise would enhance endurance performance during very prolonged exercise when depletion of body carbohydrate stores must develop (53).

The biomechanical model

A key predictor of the biomechanical model is that increased movement economy would improve performance by reducing the rate of heat accumulation during exercise. This model also explains that a reduced body mass would improve performance during prolonged exercise as it slows the rate of heat accumulation during more vigorous exercise especially when the environmental conditions are severe (19).

The importance of elastic return energy, especially in weight-bearing sports, and the identification of stretch/shortening cycle fatigue suggests that training may improve elasticity and delay stretch/shortening cycle fatigue, perhaps by altering the elastic component of skeletal muscle, tendons and ligaments.

References

1. Bale J, Sang J. *Kenyan running*. Frank Cass, London, U.K., pp. 1-209, 1996.
2. Bassett DR, Howley ET. Maximal oxygen uptake: "classical" versus "contemporary" viewpoints. *Med Sci Sports Exerc* 29: 591-603, 1997.
2a. Bassett DR, Howley ET. Limiting factors for maximum oxygen uptake: and determinants of endurance performance. *Med Sci Sports Exerc* 32: 70-84, 2000.
2b. Bergh UB, Ekblom B, Åstrand P.-O. Maximal oxygen uptake: "classical" versus "contemporary" viewpoints. *Med Sci Sports Exerc* 32: 85-88, 2000.
3. Bergstrom JB, Hermansen L, Hultman E, Saltin B. Diet, muscle glycogen and physical performance. *Acta Physiol Scand* 71: 140-150, 1967.
4. Berthon, P., Fellmann, N., Bedu, M., Beaune, B., Dabonneville, M., Coudert, J., Chamoux, A. A 5-min running field test as a measurement of maximal aerobic velocity. *Eur. J Appl Physiol* 75: 233-238, 1997.
5. Booth J, Marino F, Ward JJ. Improved running performance in hot humid conditions following whole body precooling. *Med Sci Sports Exerc* 29: 943-949, 1997.
6. Bosch AN, Dennis SC, Noakes TD. Influence of carbohydrate loading on fuel substrate turnover and oxidation during prolonged exercise. *J Appl Physiol* 74: 1921-1927, 1993.
7. Bosch AN, Goslin BR, Noakes TD, Dennis SC. Physiological differences between black and white runners during a treadmill marathon. *Europ J Appl Physiol* 61: 68-72, 1990.
8. Bosch AN, Weltan SM, Dennis SC, Noakes TD.: Fuel substrate kinetics of carbohydrate loading differs from that of carbohydrate ingestion during prolonged exercise. *Metabolism* 45: 415-423, 1996.
9. Coetzer P, Noakes TD, Sanders B, Lambert MI, Bosch AN, Wiggins I, Dennis SC. Superior fatigue resistance of elite black South African distance runners. *J Appl Physiol* 75: 1822-1827. 1993.
10. Conley DL, Krahenbuhl GS. Running economy and distance running performance of highly trained athletes. *Med Sci Sports Exerc* 12: 357-360. 1980.
11. Costill DL, Winrow E. Maximal oxygen intake among marathon runners. *Arch Phys Med Rehab* 51: 317-320. 1970a.

12. Costill DL, Winrow E. A comparison of two middle-aged ultramarathon runners. *Res Quart* 41: 135-139. 1970b.
13. Costill DL, Thomason H, Roberts E. Fractional utilization of the aerobic capacity during distance running. *Med Sci Sports Exerc* 5: 248-252. 1973.
14. Costill DL. The relationship between selected physiological variables and distance running performance. *J Sports Med Physical Fitness* 7: 61-66. 1967.
15. Costill DL. A scientific approach to distance running. *Track and Field News,* Los Altos, California, 1979.
16. Coyle EF, Coggan AR, Hemmert MK, Ivy JL. Muscle glycogen utilization during prolonged strenuous exercise when fed carbohydrate. *J Appl Physiol* 61: 165-172. 1986.
17. Davies CTM, Thompson MW. Aerobic performance of female marathon and male ultramarathon athletes. *Europ J Appl Physiol* 61: 611-617. 1979.
18. Davis JM, Bailey SP. Possible mechanisms of central nervous system fatigue during exercise. *Med Sci Sports Exerc* 29(1): 45-57. 1997.
19. Dennis SC, Noakes TD. Advantages of smaller body mass for distance running performances in warm, humid conditions. *Eur J Appl Physiol* 79: 280-284. 1999.
20. Dill DB, Talbot JH, Edwards HT. Studies in muscular activity. VI: Response of several individuals to a fixed task. *J Physiol* 69: 267-305. 1930.
21. Fitts RH, Costill DL, Gardetto PR. Effect of swim exercise training on human muscle fiber function. *J Appl Physiol* 66: 465-475. 1989.
22. Fitts RH, Widrick JJ. Muscle mechanics: adaptations with exercise-training. *Exerc Sports Sci Rev* 24: 427-473. 1996.
23. Foster C. VO_2-max and training indices as determinants of competitive running performance. *J Sports Sci* 1: 13-22. 1983.
24. Foster C, Costill DL, Daniels JT, Fink WJ. Skeletal muscle enzyme activity, fiber composition and VO_2-max in relation to distance running performance. *Europ J Appl Physiol* 39: 73-80. 1978.
25. Galloway SD, Maughan RJ. Effects of ambient temperature on the capacity to perform prolonged cycle exercise in man. *Med Sci Sports Exerc* 29: 1240-1249. 1997.
26. González-Alonso J, Teller C, Andersen SL, Jensen FB, Hyldig T, Nielsen B. Influence of body temperature on the development of fatigue during prolonged exercise in the heat. *J Appl Physiol* 86: 1032-1039. 1999.
27. Graham TE, Saltin B. Estimation of the mitochondrial redox state in human skeletal muscle during exercise. *J Appl Physiol* 66: 561-566. 1989.
28. Grant S, Craig I, Wilson J, Aitchison T. The relationship between 3 km running performance and selected physiological variables. *J Sports Sci* 15: 403-410, 1997.
29. Hill AV. *Living machinery.* G Dell and Sons Ltd, London, pp. 1-241, 1927.
30. Hill AV, Long CNH, Lupton H. Muscular exercise, lactic acid, and the supply and utilization of oxygen: parts I-III. *Proc Royal Soc Bri* 96: 438-475, 1924a.

31. Hill AV, Long CNH, Lupton H. Muscular exercise, lactic acid, and the supply and utilization of oxygen: parts IV-VI. *Proc Royal Soc Br* 97: 84-138, 1924b.

32. Hill, AV, Long CNH, Lupton H. Muscular exercise, lactic acid, and the supply and utilization of oxygen: parts VII-VIII. *Proc Roy Soc B* 97: 155-176, 1924c.

33. Hochochka, PW. The metabolic implications of intracellular circulation. *Proc Natl Acad Sci* 96: 12233-12239, 1999.

34. Jones AM, Doust JH. The validity of the lactate minimum test for determination of the maximal lactate steady state. *Med Sci Sports Exerc* 30: 1304-1313, 1998.

35. Komi PV, Nicol C. *Stretch-shortening cycle fatigue.* Biomechanics and Biology of Movement. 1998.

36. Krahenbuhl GS, Pangrazi RP. Characteristics associated with running performance in young boys. *Med Sci Sports Exerc* 5: 486-490, 1983.

37. Lacour JR, Padilla S, Barthelemy JC, Dormois D. The energetics of middle-distance running. *Eur J Appl Physiol* 60: 38-43, 1990.

38. Lacour JR, Padilla S, Chatard JCm Arsac L, Barthelemy JC. Assessment of running velocity at maximal oxygen uptake. *Eur J Appl Physiol* 62: 77-82, 1991.

39. Matsui H, Miyashita M, Kiura M, Kabayshi K, Hoshikawa T, Kamei S. Maximum oxygen intake and its relationship to body weight of Japanese adolescents. *Med Sci Sports* 3: 170-175, 1972.

40. McCann DJ, Adams WC. Wet bulb globe temperature index and performance in competitive distance runners. Med Sci Sports Exerc 29: 955-961, 1997.

41. Mitchell JH, Blomqvist G. Maximal oxygen uptake. *New Engl J Med* 284: 1018-1022, 1971.

42. Miyashita M, Miura M, Murase Y, Yamaji K. Running performance from the viewpoint of aerobic power. In: Folinsbee LJ, Wagner JA, Borgia JF, Drinkwater BL, Gliner JA, Bedi JF (eds). *Environmental stress: Individual human adaptations,* Academic Press, New York 183-194, 1978.

43. Morgan DW, Baldini FD, Martin PE, Kohrt WM. Ten kilometer performance and predicted velocity at VO_2-max among well-trained male runners. *Med Sci Sports Exerc* 21: 78-83, 1989.

44. Nicol C, Komi PV, Marconnet P. Fatigue effects of marathon running on neuromuscular performance. I. Changes in muscle force and stiffness characteristics. *Scand J Med Sci Sports* 1: 10-17, 1991.

45. Nielsen B, Hales JRS, Strange S, Christensen NJ, Warberg J, Saltin BN. Human circulatory and thermoregulatory adaptations with heat acclimatization and exercise in a hot, dry environment. *J Physiol* 460: 467-485, 1993.

46. Nielsen B, Savard G, Richter EA, Hargreaves M, Saltin B. Muscle blood flow and muscle metabolism during exercise and heat stress. *J Appl Physiol* 69: 1040-1046, 1990.

47. Nielsen B, Strange S, Christensen NJ, Warberg J, Saltin B. Acute and adaptive responses in humans to exercise in a warm, humid environment. *Pflügers Arch* 434: 49-56, 1997.

48. Noakes TD. Implications of exercise testing for prediction of athletic performance: a contemporary perspective. *Med Sci Sports Exerc* 20: 319-330, 1988.

49. Noakes TD. *Lore of Running.* Oxford University Press, Cape Town, 3rd Edition, pp. 1-535, 1992.

50. Noakes TD. Challenging beliefs: ex Africa semper aliquid novi. *Med Sci Sports Exerc* 29: 571-590, 1997.

51. Noakes TD. Maximal oxygen uptake: "classical" versus "contemporary" viewpoints. A rebuttal. *Med Sci Sports Exerc* 30(9): 1381-1398, 1998a.

52. Noakes TD. Why do Africans run so swiftly? A research challenge for African scientists. *S Afr J Sci* 94: 531-535, 1998b.

53. Noakes TD. Physiological models to understand exercise fatigue and the adaptations that predict or enhance athletic performance. *Scand J Exerc Sci Sports Med* 10: 123-145, 2000.

54. Noakes TD, Myburgh KH, Schall R. Peak treadmill running velocity during the VO_2-max test predicts running performance. *J Sports Sci* 8: 35-45, 1990.

55. Norton K, Olds T, Olive S, Craig N. Anthropometry and Sports Performance. In: K. Norton and T. Olds. *Anthropometrica,* University of New South Wales Press, pp. 289-364, 1996.

56. O'Brien MJ, Viguie CA, Mazzeo RS, Brooks GA. Carbohydrate dependence during marathon running. *Med Sci Sports Exerc* 25: 1009-1017, 1993.

57. Padilla S, Bourdin M, Barthélémy JC, Lacour JR. Physiological correlates of middle-distance running performance. *Eur J Appl Physiol* 65: 561-566, 1992.

58. Pennisi E. A new view of how leg muscles operate on the run. *Science* 275: 1067, 1997.

59. Pollock ML. Submaximal and maximal working capacity of elite distance runners, Part I: Cardiorespiratory aspects. *Ann NY Acad Sci* 301: 310-321, 1977.

60. Raskoff WJ, Goldman S, Cohn K. The "Athletic Heart". Prevalence and physiological significance of left ventricular enlargement in distance runners. *JAMA* 236: 158-162, 1976.

61. Rauch LHG, Hawley JA, Noakes TD, Dennis SC. Fuel metabolism during ultra-endurance exercise. *Pflügers Arch* 436: 211-219, 1998.

62. Richardson RS, Noyszewski EA, Leigh JS, Wagner PD. Lactate efflux from exercising human skeletal muscle: role of intracellular P. *J Appl Physiol* 85: 627-634, 1998.

63. Roberts JR, Marsh RL, Weyand PG, Taylor CR. Muscular force in running turkeys: The economy of minimizing work. *Science* 275: 1113-1115, 1997.

64. Rowell LB. *Human cardiovascular control.* Oxford University Press, New York, pp. 1-500, 1993.

65. Saltin B, Astrand P-O. Maximal oxygen uptake in athletes. *J. Appl. Physiol.* 23: 353-358, 1967.

66. Saltin B, Kim CK, Terrados N, Larsen H, Svedenhag J, Rolf C. Morphology, enzyme activities and buffer capacity in leg muscles of Kenyan and Scandinavian runners. *Scand J Med Sci Sports* 5: 222-230, 1995a.

67. Saltin B, Larsen H, Terrados N, Bangsbo J, Bak T, Kim CK, Svedenhag J, Rolf CJ. Aerobic exercise capacity at sea level and at altitude in Kenyan boys, junior and senior runners compared with Scandinavian runners. *Scand J Med Sci Sports* 5: 209-221, 1995b.

68. Saltin B. Adaptive responses to training at medium altitude; with a note on Kenyan runners and a proposal for a multi-centre study. Revised and extended version of Saltin B. Exercise and the Environment: focus on altitude. *Res Quart Exerc Sport* 67: 1-10, 1996.

69. Scott BK, Houmard JA. Peak running velocity is highly related to distance running performance. *Int J Sports Med* 15: 504-507, 1994.

70. Scrimgeour AG, Noakes TD, Adams B, Myburgh K. The influence of weekly training distance on fractional utilization of maximum aerobic capacity in marathon and ultramarathon runners. *Eur J Appl Physiol* 55: 202-209, 1986.

71. Svedenhag J, Sjodin B. Physiological characteristics of elite male runners in and of season. *Can J Appl Sport Sci* 10: 127-133, 1985.

72. Tanser T. Train hard, *Win Easy*. Tafnews Press Inc., USA, pp. 1-198, 1997.

73. Taylor CR, Lyman CP. Heat storage in running antelopes: independence of brain and body temperatures. *Am J Physiol* 22: 114-117, 1972.

74. Taylor CR, Rowntree VJ. Temperature regulation and heat balance in running cheetahs: a strategy for sprinters? *Amer J Physiol* 224: 848-851, 1973.

75. Taylor HL, Buskirk E, Henschel A. Maximal oxygen intake as an objective measure of cardio-respiratory performance. *J Appl Physiol* 8: 73-80, 1955.

76. Weston A.R., Karamizrak, O., Smith, A., Noakes, T.D., Myburgh K.H. African runners exhibit greater fatigue resistance, lower lactate accumulation, and higher oxidative enzyme activity. *J. Appl. Physiol.* 86: 915-923, 1999.

77. Wyndham CH, Strydom NB, van Rensburg AJ, Benade AJS. Physiological requirements for world-class performances in endurance running. *S Afr Med J* 43: 996-1002, 1969.

78. Yoshida T, Udo M, Iwai K, Yamaguchi T. Physiological characteristics related to endurance running performance in female distance runners. *J. Sports Sci* 11L 57-62, 1993.

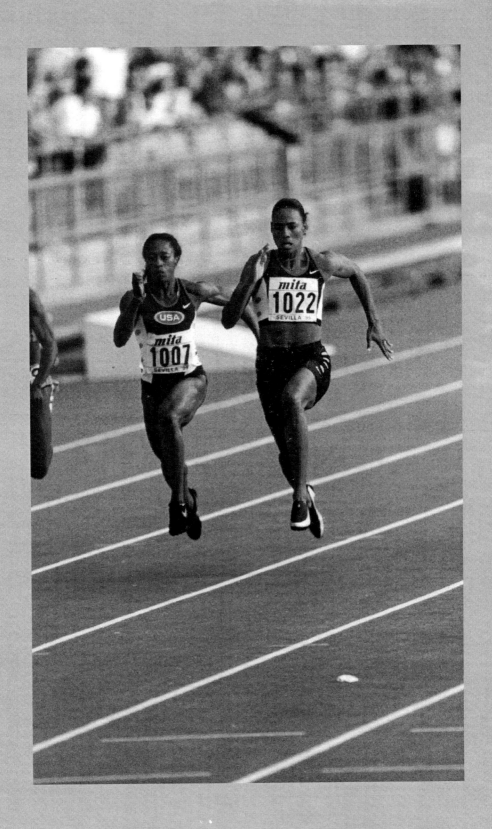

Muscle Fibre Type Characteristics of the Runner

Jesper L. Andersen

Synopsis

This chapter reviews the fibre type composition in skeletal muscles of elite endurance-, middle distance-, and sprint-runners. The possible significance of the fibre type composition for optimal performance in endurance- and sprint-running is evaluated. Furthermore, based on a number of new exercise-training studies, a hypothetical proposal of how the fibre type (myosin heavy chain isoform) composition may change during a yearly training circle in the skeletal muscles of an elite sprinter is provided.

Introduction

Runners are as different as humans are in general, ranging from the skinny marathon-runner to the brawny sprinter. Consequently, a description of the muscle fibre type characteristics of a runner is not an unambiguous deed, but rather a summation of different muscle compositions reflecting the distinct specialisation seen in today's top runners.

The term „runner" is most often associated with more endurance-like performance. Likewise, data on middle- and long-distance runners are much more numerous than data on sprint-runners. In the following I will review differences in muscle fibre type composition between different categories of runners and, in addition, focus on the muscle fibre composition of sprinters and the ability of specific training para-

49

digms to alter the muscle fibre composition towards a composition that favours short-distance sprint-running.

Based on traditional ATPase histochemistry human skeletal muscle fibres can be divided into the slow type 1, and the fast type 2a and 2b fibres (9). The literature reveals that the human skeletal muscle most commonly examined – the vastus lateralis – in long-distance runners

Table 1. Summary of published values of fibre type distribution in m. vastus lateralis and gastrocnemius of middle- and long-distance runners

Reference	Fibre type in %			Sex	No.	Mu.	Category of runner and comments
	1	2a	2b				
Parkhouse et al., 1985 (30)[N,*]	43	58	-	-	5	V	800-m runners (PB, 800 m <1.55 min.)†
Denis et al., 1992 (11)[N,*]	58	42	-	M	8	V	800-m runners (PB, 800m; 1,51 min) (A; type 1: 53%)
Gregor et al., 1981 (18)[A,*]	56	44	-	W	7	V	800-m/distance runners (PB, 800m: 2,09 min.)
Gollnick et al., 1972 (16)[N,*]	51	49	-	M	2	V	middle-distance (US elite) (A; type 1: 49%)
Boros-Hatfaludy et al., 1986 (8)[N,*]	60	40	-	M	6	V	middle-distance (800-5000 m runners)
Howald, 1982 (24)[N]	63	35	2	-	7	V	middle-distance ("best Swiss 800-1500 m runners)
Gregor et al., 1979 (17)[A,*]	63	37	-	M	9	V	"middle-distance"
Saltin et al., 1995 (37)[N]	64	32	4	M/W	12	V	middle-distance (Scandinavian elite)
Saltin et al., 1995 (37)[N]	65	31	4	M	9	V	middle-distance (Kenyan junior elite)
Saltin et al., 1995 (37)[N]	72	25	3	M	4	V	middle-distance (Kenyan elite)
Gregor et al., 1981 (18)[A,*]	73	27	-	W	7	V	middle-distance (US elite)
Torok et al., 1995 (46)[N]	65	32	3	M	6	V	middle and long distance (PB, 5000m: <16.45 min)
Tesch & Karlsson, 1985 (43)[N,*]	67	33	-	M	9	V	middle and long distance (A; type 1: 67%)
Howald, 1982 (24)[N]	78	20	2	M	9	V	"long-distance" ("best Swiss 5000m-marathon runners)
Sadoyama et al., 1988 (34)[A,*]	64	36	-	M	7	V	"distance-runners"
Johansson et al., 1987 (26)[N]	59	33	8	M	5	V	"marathon-runners" (PB, marathon: 2.36 h)
Gollnick et al., 1972 (16)[N,*]	73	27	-	M	2	V	"distance" (US elite) (A; type 1: 71%)
Gregor et al., 1979 (17)[A,*]	73	27	-	M	4	V	"long distance"
Thorstensson et al., 1977 (45)[N,*]	67	33	-	M	7	V	orienteers (Swedish elite)
Jansson & Kaijser, 1977 (25)[N]	70	27	3	M	8	V	orienteers (Swedish elite)
Rolf et al., 1997 (33)[N]	73	27	0	M	5	V	Swedish elite orienteers ("world class"), (VO_2max:79)

Rolf et al., 1997 (33) [N]	79	21	0	W	7	V	Swedish elite orienteers ("world class"), (VO$_2$max: 68)
Costill et al., 1976 (10) [N,*]	52	48	-	F	7	G	PB 800 m: 2.08,1 min
Costill et al., 1976 (10) [N,*]	61	39	-	M	7	G	PB 800 m: 1.51,5 min
Boros-Hatfaludy et al., 1986 (8) [N,*]	59	41	-	M	6	G	middle-distance (800-5000 m runners)
Saltin et al., 1977 (36) [N]	62	37	1	M	10	G	"Runners"
Fink et al., 1977 (13) [N,*]	62	38	-	M	18	G	"Good middle distance runners"
Farrell et al., 1979 (12) [N,*]	64	36	-	M	18	G	"distance runners" (VO$_2$max: 62)
Costill et al., 1976 (10) [N,*]	69	31	-	M	5	G	"Distance runners" (PB marathon, 5000m: 2.44 h, 14.09 min)
Jansson & Kaijser, 1977 (25) [N]	68	30	2	M	7	G	orienteers (Swedish elite)
Rolf et al., 1997 (33) [N]	68	32	1	W	7	G	Swedish elite orienteers ("world class"), (VO$_2$max: 68)
Rolf et al., 1997 (33) [N]	71	27	1	M	5	G	Swedish elite orienteers ("world class"), (VO$_2$max:79)
Fink et al., 1977 (13) [N,*]	79	21	-	M	14	G	"Elite distance runners"

*; only ST/FT (type 1/type 2) is presented in the original paper, No.; Number of subjects, Mu.; Muscle, N; fibre type distribution in relative number(%), A; fibre type distribution in area percentage, M; men, W; women, V; vastus lateralis, G; gastrocnemius, BP; average best performance for the group, on the specified distance, VO$_2$max: Maximal oxygen uptake in ml•min^{-1}•kg^{-1}. †; in the original paper these subjects are categorised as "sprinters".

contains approximately 75% type 1, 25% type 2a, and no or only a few percent type 2b fibres (Table 1). In comparison, middle-distance runners demonstrate somewhat less type 1, and more type 2a and to some extent also type 2b fibres (11, 18, 35, 37) (Table 1). The average fibre type composition of successful sprinters seems to be opposite of that of the long-distance runners, i.e. 30% type 1, 50% type 2a and 20% type 2b fibres (Table 2). It should be emphasised that large variations can be observed between individuals in the three categories.

Recent findings indicate that the separation into three different fibre types on the basis of ATPase histochemistry may be too simplistic, and also to some extent misleading, at least when certain groups of athletes are concerned (4, 5, 20). Myosin, the contractile protein of the thick filament, has been shown to be the key determinant regulating the shortening properties of the skeletal muscle fibres (20, 38). Furthermore, besides being directly linked to the shortening properties of the skeletal muscle fibre, the presence of a specific myosin isoform is also a valuable marker for other fibre type-specific features such as metabolic profile and fatigue characteristics (31, 32). Under steady-state conditions certain metabolic properties including the relative amount of myoglobin and number of mitochondria as well as activity of a num-

Table 2. Summary of some published values of fibre type distribution in m. vastus lateralis of sprint-runners

Fibre types (%)

Reference	1	2a	2b	Sex	No.	Mu.	Category of runner and comments
Gollnick et al., 1972 (16)[N,*]	26	74	-	M	1	V	sprinter (PB 100 yd: 9.3 s), (A; type 1; 22%)
Johansson et al., 1987 (26)[N]	30	43	27	M	5	V	sprinters (PB, 100m: 10.9 s)
Sadoyama et al.,1988 (34)[A,*]	30	70	-	M	12	V	"sprinters"
Mero et al., 1981 (29)[A]	32	40	28	M	4	V	"Finnish sprinters", (PB, 100m: 10.7 s)
Mero et al., 1981 (29)[A]	37	37	26	M	7	V	"Finnish sprinters" (PB, 100m: 11.1 s)
Gregor et al., 1979 (17)[N,*]	39	61	-	W	3	V	"sprinters"
Thorstensson et al., 1977 (45)[N,*]	39	61	-	M	9	V	"sprinters" (Swedish elite) (S/J)
Fridén et al., 1988 (14)[N]	39	37	24	M	6	V	(PB, 200 m: 22.8 s)
Gregor et al., 1981 (18)[A,*]	41	59	-	W	2	V	"sprinters" (US elite)
Hirvonen et al., 1987 (22)[N,*]	40	60	-	M	7	V	"Finnish sprinters" (PR, 100m: 10.89 s)
Denis et al., 1992 (11)[N,*]	41	59	-	M	8	V	"sprinters" (PB, 100m: 10.6 s) (A: type 1; 36%)
Andersen et al, 1994 (5)[N]	43	47	10	M	6	V	"sprinters" (PB, 100m: 10.89 s)
Torok et al., 1995 (46)[N]	46	47	7	M	6	V	"sprinters" (PB, <11.1 s on 100 m)
Boros-Hatfaludy et al., 1986 (8)[N,*]	46	53	-	M	7	V	"sprinters"
Bauman et al., 1987 (7)[N]	49	41	10	M	8	V	"sprinters"
Mero et al., 1981 (29)[A]	51	31	18	M	6	V	"Finnish sprinters" (PR, 100m: 11.5 s)
Costill et al., 1976 (10)[N,*]	27	73	-	F	2	G	"sprinters" (PB, 100m: 11.4 s)
Costill et al., 1976 (10)[N,*]	24	76	-	M	2	G	"sprinters" (PB, 100m: 10.5 s)
Boros-Hatfaludy et al., 1986 (8)[N,*]	57	43	-	M	7	G	"sprinters"

*: only ST/FT (type 1/type 2) is presented in the original paper, No.; Number of subjects, Mu.; Muscle. N; fibre type distribution in relative number (%), A; fibre type distribution in area percentage. M; men, W; women, V; vastus lateralis, G; gastrocnemius, BP; average best performance for the group on the specified distance, S/J; sprinters and jumpers.

ber of glycolytic (e.g. lactate dehydrogenase) and oxidative (e.g. malate dehydrogenase) enzymes can be assigned to the different MHC-based fibre type populations (32) (Table 3). Although, during shifts in training pattern or intensity this close coupling might be altered (32). For example, enzyme activities of aerobic-oxidative metabolic pathways may increase in exercising muscle without noticeable MHC-based fibre type transitions (31). The adult human skeletal muscles expresses three different isoforms of the *M*yosin *H*eavy *C*hain protein; MHC I, MHC IIA and MHC IIX (38). Ideally, type 1 fibres contain MHC I, type 2a fibres MHC IIA and type 2b fibres MHC IIX (Table 3), but

Table 3. Functional and metabolic characteristics of human skeletal muscle fibre types

Fibre types	MHC isoform content	Functional characteristics	Metabolic characteristics
1	MHC I	Long time to peak tension Low maximal unloaded shortening velocity Low rate of force development High fatigue resistance	Low glycogenolytic enzyme activity High mitochondrial enzyme activity
2a	MHC 2A	Short time to peak tension Higher maximal unloaded shortening velocity Higher rate of force development Lower fatigue resistance	High glycogenolytic enzyme activity Medium mitochondrial enzyme activity
2b	MHC 2X	Shortest time to peak tension Highest maximal unloaded shortening velocity Highest rate of force development Lowest fatigue resistance	High glycogenolytic enzyme activity Low mitochondrial enzyme activity

thorough examination of the MHC content of single human skeletal muscle fibres has revealed that a considerable number of fibres in fact contain two different MHC isoforms (3, 4, 5, 27, 28). This phenomenon; the MHC isoform co-expression, may be especially pronounced in muscles from certain athletes, or in athletes markedly increasing or decreasing their amount/type of training (3, 5). Thus, a group of elite sprint-runners had 15% type 2b fibres as determined by ATPase histochemistry, whereas the single fibres analysis of the same biopsies revealed that only 0.1% of the fibres contained solely MHC IIX. Consequently, in the vastus laterlis muscle of these sprint-runners only 1 out of each 150 histochemically determined type 2b fibres contained solely MHC IIX, the remaining 149 „type 2b" fibres co-expressed varying amounts of MHC IIX and MHC IIA (3, 5).

Although training for long-distance running utilises both long and short training-cycles, it requires a training-schedule with a constantly high amount of fairly uniform endurance-like running. Training for sprint-distances does, on a yearly basis, include much greater variation in the amount and types of training. Therefore, when a long-distance runner after years of conducting endurance-like running, has reached a certain high level of training intensity and cannot tolerate a further addition in the amount of training conducted, it is likely that he or she will not show great variations in muscle MHC isoform expression on a yearly basis. Recent results seem to indicate that this is not the case for elite sprint-runners (5).

All kinds of physical activity seem to reduce the expression of the fastest MHC isoform (2, 5, 15), whereas detraining has the opposite effect (3, 41), suggesting that the MHC IIX constitutes the „default" MHC gene (3, 6, 15, 20). When planning a sprinter's training-schedule this notion would favour a period of reduced training leading up to a major competition event. In fact, a typical sprinter has a long preparation period including large amounts of heavy resistance-training defined as relatively few near-maximal muscle contractions against a heavy external load and short interval-running, whereas in the competition period only limited amounts of short fast-running, explosive and dynamic training exercises, and technical drills will be engaged. We have evidence that a period of increased heavy-resistance training (as conducted by sprinters) will decrease the expression of MHC IIX, but more interestingly, if this is followed by a period of detraining, the expression of MHC IIX will be boosted to levels even higher than those observed prior to heavy-resistance training (3). Furthermore, we have examined muscle biopsies from a group of elite sprinters before and after a 3 month period of combined heavy-resistance training and short interval-running. Results from this study have lead to the suggestion of the so-called bi-directional switch in MHC expression (MHC I → MHC IIA ← MHC IIX) (Figure 1). These data suggest the possibility of the complex activity pattern conducted in sprint-training resulting in, not only a significant shift in expression between MHC IIA and MHC IIX but also a shift in expression between MHC I and MHC IIA.

If, on the other hand, it is hypothesised that all types of physical activity reduce expression of the MHC IIX isoform and that all muscle activity pushes the MHC expression, not only in the direction: MHC IIX → MHC IIA, but also in the direction: MHC IIA → MHC I (40), it becomes very difficult to conduct physical exercise training that leads towards a decrease in the proportion of type 1 fibres. Therefore, another strategy for the sprint athlete to obtain a relatively high amount of fast MHC in his or her muscles, could be to increase the cross-sectional area of the already existing type 2 fibres, without affecting the type 1 fibres (at least to the same extend), leading to a faster contracting muscle (1). This is actually what happens with heavy-resistance training, type 2 fibres hypertrophy more than type 1 fibres (3, 19, 21, 23, 35, 42, 44).

„The bi-directional transformation of MHC isoforms"

MHC I $\rightarrow$ MHC IIA $\leftarrow$ MHC IIX (sprint training)

"The uni-directional transformation of MHC isoforms"

MHC I $\rightarrow$ MHC IIA $\longrightarrow$ MHC IIX (decreased training activity)

MHC I $\leftarrow$ MHC IIA $\longleftarrow$ MHC IIX (increased training activity)

Figure 1. The bi-directional transformation is probably a product of a true fibre type transition, as revealed by the histochemical data and the analysis of MHC composition of single fibres (5). Furthermore, this process is fortified by a tendency towards a difference in hypertrophy of the fibre types, so that type 2 fibres shows more hypertrophy than type 1 fibres, if subjected to heavy-resistance training. Both of these processes will lead in the direction of a higher relative amount of MHC II in the muscles of the sprinter. Included in the figure is the "uni-directional" transformation, that constitutes the conventional shift in MHC isoform expression in consequence of training/detraining (40).

An interesting finding regarding differences in fibre size between the fibre types in runners has been reported by Sjöström et al. (39). They found that the fibre sizes of the three main fibre types in the vastus lateralis muscle of a group of marathon runners were almost identical (type 1; 4800 μm^2, type 2a; 4500 μm^2 and type 2b; 4600 μm^2), whereas the average fibre sizes from a group of sprinters showed distinct differences among the different fibre types type (type 1; 5000 μm^2, type 2a; 7300 μm^2 and type 2b; 5900 μm^2). We have results from a group of sprinters (5) that are very similar to those published by Sjöström et al. (39). In our group of sprinters the fibre sizes were: Type 1; 5000 μm^2, type 2a; 6300 μm^2 and type 2b; 5400 μm^2 (Andersen, not previously published data). These results indicate that the type of training conducted by sprinters, in contrast to the type of training conducted by long-distance runners, gives rise to a selective hypertrophy specifically located in the type 2a fibres as proposed above. For a more detailed description of the possible differences between evaluating „fibre type composition" as to relative percentage of fibre type, relative area percentage of the fibre types or the relative MHC isoform composition, see Figure 2.

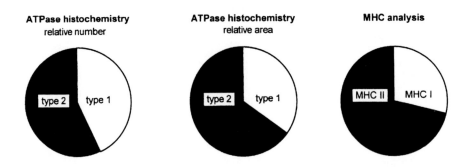

Figure 2. Caution should be taken when comparing fibre type composition data from different studies (as those presented in tables 1 and 2). The actual method of evaluation can be crucial for the percentages obtained, at least for certain subjects. Thus, using ATPase histochemistry the average fibre type composition of m. vastus lateralis in a group of elite sprinters was found to be 43% type 1 fibres and 57% type 2 fibres (relative numbers). The fibre area percentage was 35% type 1 fibres and 65% type 2 fibres. When the same biopsies were examined for actual MHC I composition they were found to contain only 29% MHC I and 71% MHC II (relative percentages) (Andersen, not previously published data). Therefore, it is not uncommon to observe that a biopsy from m. vastus lateralis from a sprinter contains 35% type 1 fibres, but due to the difference in size of type 1 and type 2 fibres the actual content of MHC I in the biopsy is only 20-25%. These considerable variations cover the fact that the type 2 muscle fibres of the sprint-runner through extensive heavy resistance-training has hypertrophied more than the type 1 fibres, resulting in a larger difference in size between type 1 and type 2 fibres than is observed in endurance-trained runners and untrained subjects. Therefore, one will often find higher resemblances between methods of conducting fibre type evaluation in endurance-runners, than in runners engaged in heavy resistance-training.

On the basis of the above mentioned data and along with knowledge of the seasonal variation in the training pattern, a hypothetical model could be proposed for the MHC isoform changes that occur in the muscles of sprinters competing on a high level. Thus, it is suggested that the seasonal variations in training load and pattern will facilitate a corresponding „oscillation" of the MHC isoform expression in the muscles of the sprinter (Figure 3). The postulated MHC oscillation rests upon the assumption that the relative expression of MHC I only changes slightly with normal physical training, at least of a non-endurance like nature, whereas the main alterations in MHC expression definitely occur between the MHC IIA and MHC IIX isoforms, which seem to mirror each others relative expression at all times during the yearly circle.

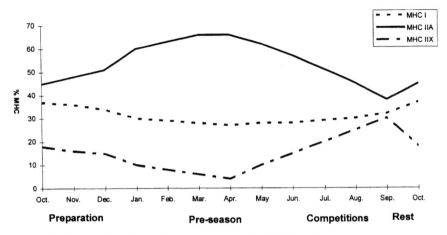

Oscillations in relative MHC isoform expression in muscles of Sprinters

Figure 3. A hypothetical model suggesting how the MHC isoform expression may „oscillate" in the skeletal muscles of a typical sprint runner, during a one year training cycle, in response to the various amount and types of training performed. For further details and explanation see text.

An oscillation in the MHC expression, like the one proposed to occur in the skeletal muscles of the sprinter, would not be expected to take place in the muscles of long-distance runners during a yearly training circle, due to their constantly high amount of fairly uniform endurance-like running. Furthermore, if a phenomenon such as „muscle memory" exists (41) it is likely that the muscles of the sprinters, which are accustomed to frequent and rapid changes in training patterns, will react more promptly upon the variations in training pattern and loading, than the muscles of the long-distance runner exposed to a hard invariant tonic type of training.

As mentioned above, heavy-resistance training seems to evoke a significant decrease in the expression of MHC IIX, and most likely this holds true for long-term endurance-training as well (20). But how will fast-pace running of a more interval-like nature, the kind of training conducted by long-sprinters and those running the shorter middle-distances, affect MHC expression? In a recent study we subjected six young men to three months of heavy-resistance training. Prior to entering the heavy-resistance training period the six subjects were homogeneous in the sense that they had matching $\dot{V}O_2$-max, general activity level, and performed equally well in a number of strength-related tests, but three subjects had a „naturally" low relative expression of MHC IIX in their vastus lateralis muscle, and three of the subjects had a „naturally" high relative expression of MHC IIX in their vastus lateralis muscle. In all subjects, whether they had a high or a low relative expression of MHC IIX to begin with, the heavy-resistance training resulted in an almost complete disappearance of MHC IIX expression in the trained muscles. After this period of resistance-training the subjects abruptly switched exercise pattern and performed two months of training consisting of only short interval-running, corresponding to the training conducted by sprinters in their pre-season preparation. Interestingly, the individual subgroups of subjects responded differently to this shift in activity pattern (Figure 4). The subjects, who had small amounts of MHC IIX expression prior to entering the heavy-resistance training period, showed only minor variations, in the MHC IIX expression, from the untrained state, in response to the heavy-resistance training and interval-running periods (Figure 4). On the contrary, the subjects who had a high relative proportion of MHC IIX prior to resistance training, experienced an almost total disappearance of the MHC IIX expression in the trained muscle, or in other terms; the MHC IIX was „trained away". But interestingly, following the rather hard and exhausting interval-running program, their muscles were not able to „maintain" the very low MHC IIX expression that had appeared as a consequence of the heavy-resistance training. Thus, during the interval-running period, the expression of MHC IIX in the vastus lateralis muscle of these three subjects almost returned to the pre-resistance training level. A conclusion from this experiment is, that apparently heavy-resistance training is a more potent stimulus than short interval-running for suppressing MHC IIX expression. Based on the different responses to the training, the subjects could be divided into two distinct subgroups; the „responders" and the „non-responders" (Figure 4). This suggestion of potential „responders" and „non-responders" may also, at least in part explain why some athletes tend to respond well to interval training, whereas others do not respond so well.

Bearing the above in mind, it is reasonable to suggest that the initial (probably inherited) MHC isoform composition of an adult individual's muscles could be important for the response to a given training stimulus. Further along this chain of thought, it would seem difficult to expect

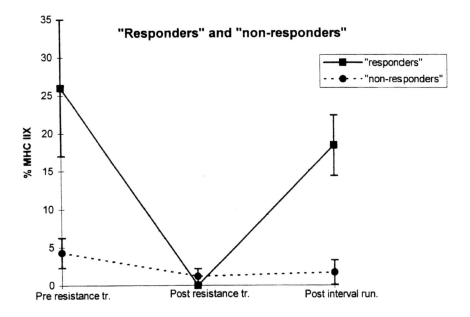

Figure 4. Data of six subjects, who performed three months of heavy resistance-trai-ning, and then switched to two months of sprint interval-running consisting of 3-4 series of 3-4 runs of 150-250 m at near maximal speed, 3 times a week (3). Muscle biopsies were obtained before and after the heavy resistance-training period, and again after the interval-running period. As seen in the figure the subjects could be divided into two distinct groups; the „responders" (n=3) and the „non-responders" (n=3), according to differences in the potential of their muscles for responding to the different training types, by changing MHC IIX expression.

Note also that heavy resistance-training seems to be a more potent stimulus for suppressing the MHC IIX expression in the „responder"-group, than the interval-running. Both the „responders" and the „non-responders" had a 6% increase in VO_2-max after the interval-running period, compared to values obtained prior to and after resistance-training. Values are mean±SE.

that a person with a „naturally" high MHC I expression and low MHC IIX expression would easily enter into the postulated MHC isoform „oscillation" argued above. Moreover, the asserted bi-directional MHC transformation might only be a „privilege" for subjects with a certain initial MHC composition subjected to a specific activity pattern.

It is generally difficult to foresee accurately what the „optimum" fibre type composition of a top-runner, on any distance, might be, due to the difficulties of obtaining biopsies from world class runners. This becomes obvious when the performance data of the subjects involved in the studies summarised in Tables 1 and 2 are examined more closely. It appears that some of the subjects are unable, or only just able, to be part of their countries national elite in the distance in which they are competing. However, on a number of occasions it has been possible to obtain biopsies from runners of, or close to, world class standard (16, 37), but these sparse biopsies were nearly always obtained off-season, or during periods in which the runners were preparing for the competition season, and not within the narrow time range during which the world class runners were actually peaking. This means that we have limited knowledge of the fibre type composition of world class runners at their best.

A correlation between high amount of type 2 fibres and personal best time on the 100 m distance has been shown in a group of well-trained Finnish sprinters (29), but just how important the fibre type composition is for the performance of a runner we do not know. What we do know is, that the MHC composition of human skeletal muscle relates to the force and torque generation during fast joint movements (1). On the other hand, it would probably be a gross overstatement to claim that there is a straight forward correlation between the MHC composition of a runner's muscles and his or her running performance. Nevertheless, the MHC composition of e.g. m. vastus lateralis of a normal „untrained" person might give some indications of whether this person should pursue a career as a sprinter, a middle-distance, or a long-distance runner (Figure 5). A closer examination of Tables 1 and 2 reveals that top performance in a certain distance seems to require a fibre type composition within certain limits. It may be difficult to define exactly what the optimal MHC composition is for a sprinter, but undoubtfully a high amount of MHC II seems essential in the development of a world class sprinter. In broad terms a muscle composition of more than 65-75% type II fibres in m. vastus lateralis seems a necessity for a top sprinter. It is more unclear what the „optimal" MHC IIA/MHC IIX ratio is. Furthermore, as suggested earlier, the MHC IIA/IIX ratio is probably very sensitive to muscle activity and probably „oscillates" on a yearly basis, at least in some subjects. Apparently, a high class middle-distance runner must have a fibre type composition with slightly more MHC I than MHC IIA, and only small amounts of MHC IIX. An elite marathon runner should probably have a fibre type composition with a high amount of MHC I (>70%) and very little or no MHC IIX expression.

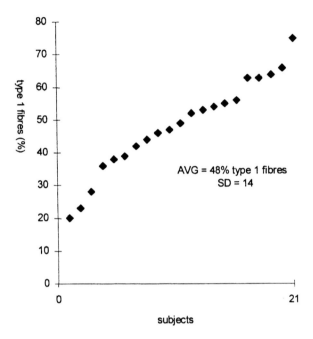

Number of type 1 fibres (%)
in vastus lateralis

Figure 5. Number of type 1 fibres, as determined by ATPase histochemistry, in m. vastus lateralis of 21sedentary young male subjects, who volunteered to participate in an exercise training study. Note that the average value of 48 % type 1 fibres covers a wide range of variation, ranging from 20% up to 75% type 1 fibres (Andersen, not previously published data). Since the daily activity level was fairly similar among the subjects, the data suggest that the genetic variation is considerable. Extrapolated to performance at a given running distance, it seems as if some subjects, due to their genetic background of having either few or many type 1 fibres, possess the potential to perform optimally on either short or long running distances (see also 36).

In conclusion, it is reasonable to claim that the long distance runner would benefit from a high amount of type 1 fibres, whereas the sprint-runner would benefit from a high amount of type 2 fibres. Today, the general belief is that training within a „normal" physical set-up only to some extent induces a shift in MHC expression from MHC II to MHC I (or vice versa), whereas a shift in expression between MHC IIA and MHC IIX is fairly easy to induce in man (3, 5, 20). Therefore, undoubtfully, successful top-runners, no matter whether they compete in long or short distances must have a suitable genetic background, determining their specific defaulted MHC isoform composition, that benefits the type of running that they are involved in.

References

1. Aagaard, P., and Andersen, J.L. Correlation between contractile strength and myosin heavy chain isoform composition in human skeletal muscle. *Med. Sci. Sports Exerc.,* 30, 1217-1222, 1998.
2. Adams, G.R., Hather, B.M., Baldwin, K.M., and Dudley, G.A. Skeletal muscle myosin heavy chain composition and resistance training. *J. Appl. Physiol.* 74, 911-915, 1993.
3. Andersen, J.L. Plasticity of myosin heavy chain isoforms in human skeletal muscle, Effects of training and detraining. Ph.D. -thesis, Dept. Human Physiol. August Krogh Inst., Copenhagen Muscle Research Centre, University of Copenhagen, Denmark, 1997.
4. Andersen, J.L., Klitgaard, H. Bangsbo, J., and Saltin B. Myosin heavy chain isoforms in single fibres from m. vastus lateralis of soccer players: Effects of strength-training. *Acta Physiol. Scand.* 150, 21-26, 1994.
5. Andersen, J.L., Klitgaard, H., and Saltin B. Myosin heavy chain isoforms in single fibres from m. vastus lateralis of sprinters: Influence of training. *Acta Physiol. Scand.* 151, 135-142, 1994.
6. Andersen, J.L., Mohr, T., Biering-Sørensen, F., Galbo H., and Kjær, M. Myosin heavy chain isoform transformation in single fibres from m. vastus lateralis in spinal cord injured individuals: effects of long-term functional electrical stimulation (FES). *Pflügers Arch.* 431, 513-518, 1996.
7. Baumann, H., Jäggi, M., Soland, F., Howald, H., and Schaub, M.C. Exercise training induces transitions of myosin isoforms subunits within histochemically typed human muscle fibres. *Pflügers Arch.,* 409, 349-360, 1987.
8. Boros-Hatfaludy, S., Fekete, G., and Apor, P. Metabolic enzyme activity patterns in muscle biopsy samples in different athletes. *Eur. J. Appl. Physiol.* 55, 334-338, 1986.
9. Brook, M.H., and Kaiser, K.K.. Three 'myosin ATPase' systems: The nature of their pH lability and sulfhydryl dependence. *J. Histochem. Cytochem.* 18, 670-672, 1970.
10. Costill, D.L., Daniels, J., Evans, W., Fink, W., Krahenbuhl, G. and Saltin, B. Skeletal muscle enzymes and fiber composition in male and female track athletes. *J. Appl. Physiol.,* 40, 149-154, 1976.
11. Denis, C., Linossier, M.T., Dormois, D., Padilla, S., Geyssant, A., Lacour, J.R., and Inbar, O. Power and metabolic responses during supramaximal exercise in 100-m and 800-m runners. *Scand. J. Med. Sci. Sports,* 2, 62-69, 1992.
12. Farrell, P.A., Wilmore, J.H., Coyle, E.F., Billing, J.E., and Costill, D.L. Plasma lactate accumulation and distance running performance. *Med. Sci. Sports,* 11, 388-344, 1979.

13. Fink, W.J., Costill, D.L., and Pollock, M.L. Submaximal and maximal working capacity of elite distance runners. Part II. Muscle fiber composition and enzyme activities. *Ann. NY Acad. Sci.* 301, 323-327, 1977.

14. Fridén, J., Seger, J, and Ekblom, B. Sublethal muscle fibre injuries after high-tension anaerobic exercise. *Eur. J. Appl. Physiol.* 57, 360-368, 1988.

15. Goldspink, G., Scutt, A., Martindale, J., Jaenicke, T., Turay, L., and Garlach, G.F. Stretch and force generation induce rapid hypertrophy and myosin isoform gene switching in adult skeletal muscle. *Biochem. Soc. Trans.* 19, 368-373, 1991.

16. Gollnick, P.D., Armstrong, R.B., Saubert, C.W., Piehl, K., and Saltin, B. Enzyme activity and fiber composition in skeletal muscle of untrained and trained men. *J. Appl. Physiol.* 33, 312-319, 1972.

17. Gregor, R.J., Edgerton, V.R., Perrine, J.J., Campion, D.S., and DeBus, C. Torque-velocity relationship and muscle fiber composition in elite female athletes. *J. Appl. Physiol.* 47, 388-392, 1979.

18. Gregor, R.J., Edgerton, V.R., Rozenek, R, and, Castleman, K.R. Skeletal muscle properties and performance in elite female track athletes. *Eur. J. Appl. Physiol.* 47, 355-364, 1981.

19. Häkkinen, K., Alén, M., and Komi, P.V. Changes in isometric force- and relaxation-time, electromyographic and muscle fibre characteristics of human skeletal muscle during strength training and detraining. *Acta Physiol. Scand.* 125, 573-585, 1985.

20. Harridge, S.D.R. The muscle contractile system and its adaptation to training. In; Human muscular function during dynamic exercise. Ed; P. Marconnet, B. Saltin, P. Komi, and J. Poortmans. *Med. Sports Sci. Basel.* 41, 82-94, 1996.

21. Hather, B.M., Tesch, P.A., Buchanan, P., and, Dudley, G.A. Influence of eccentric actions on skeletal muscle adaptations to resistance training. *Acta Physiol. Scand.* 143, 177-185, 1991.

22. Hirvonen, J., Rehunen, S., Rusko, H., and Härkönen, M. Breakdown of high-energy phosphate compounds and lactate accumulation during short supra maximal exercise. *Eur. J. Appl. Physiol.* 56, 253-259, 1987.

23. Houston, M.E., Froese, E.A., Valeriote, St.P., Green, H.J. and, Ranney, D.A. Muscle performance, morphology and metabolic capacity during strength training and detraining: a one leg model. *Eur. J. Appl. Physiol.* 51, 25-35, 1983.

24. Howald, H. Training-induced morphological and functional changes in skeletal muscle. *Int. J. Sports Med.* 3, 1-12, 1982

25. Jansson, E. and Kaijser, L. Muscle adaptation to extreme endurance training in man. *Acta Physiol. Scand.* 100, 315-324, 1977.

26. Johansson, C., Lorentzon, R., Sjöström, M., Fagerlund, M., and Fugl-Meyer, A.R. Sprinters and marathon runners. Does isokinetic knee extensor performance reflect muscle size and structure? *Acta Physiol. Scand.*, 130, 663-669, 1987.

27. Klitgaard, H., Bergman, O., Betto, R., Salviati, G., Schiaffino, S., Clausen, T., and Saltin, B. Co-existence of myosin heavy chain I and IIa isoforms in

human skeletal muscle fibres with endurance training. *Pflügers Arch.* 416, 470-472,1990.

28. Kiltgaard, H., Zhou, M., Schiaffino, S., Betto, R., Salviati, G., and Saltin, B. Ageing alters the myosin heavy chain composition of single fibres from human skeletal muscle. *Acta Physiol. Scand.* 140, 55-62, 1990.

29. Mero, A., Luhtanen, P., Viitasalo, J.T., and Komi, P.V. Relationships between the maximal running velocity, muscle fiber characteristics, force production and force relaxation of sprinters. *Scand. J. Sports Sci.* 3, 16-22, 1981.

30. Parkhouse, W.S., McKenzie, D.C., Hochachka, P.W., and Ovalle, W.K. Buffering capacity of deproteinized human vastus lateralis muscle. *J. Appl. Physiol.,* 58, 14-17, 1985.

31. Pette, D. Training effects on the contractile apparatus. *Acta Physiol. Scand.* 162, 367-376, 1998.

32. Pette, D. and Staron, R.S. Mammalian skeletal muscle fiber type transitions. *Int. Rev. Cytol.* 170, 143-223, 1997.

33. Rolf, C., Andersson, G., Westblad, P., and Saltin, B. Aerobic and anaerobic work capacities and leg muscle characteristics in elite orienteers. *Scand. J. Med. Sci. Sports,* 7, 20-24, 1997.

34. Sadoyama, T., Masuda, T., Miyata, H., and Katsuta, S. Fibre conduction velocity and fibre composition in human vastus lateralis. *Eur. J. Appl. Physiol.,* 57, 767-771, 1988.

35. Saltin, B., and Gollnick, P.D. Skeletal muscle adaptability: Significance for metabolism and performance. In; Handbook of Physiology. Section 10: Skeletal muscle. Ed; L.D. Peachey. Bethesda. *Am. Physiol. Soc.* 555-631, 1983.

36. Saltin, B., Henriksson, J., Nygaard, E., Andersen, P., and Jansson, E. Fiber types and metabolic potentials of skeletal muscles in sedentary man and endurance runners. *Ann. NY Acad. Sci.* 301, 3-29, 1977.

37. Saltin , B., Kim, C.K., Terrados, N., Larsen, H., Svedenhag, J., and Rolf, C.J. Morphology, enzyme activities and buffer capacity in leg muscles of Kenyan and Scandinavian runners. *Scand. J. Med. Sci. Sports,* 5, 222-230, 1995.

38. Schiaffino, S. and Reggiani, C. Molecular diversity of myofibrillar proteins: Gene regulation and functional significance. *Physiol. Rev.* 76, 371-423, 1996.

39. Sjöström, M., Johansson, C., and Lorentzon, R. Muscle pathmorphology in m. quadriceps of marathon runners. Early signs of stain disease or functional adaptation? *Acta Physiol. Scand.* 132, 537-542, 1988.

40. Staron, R.S., and Johnson, P. Myosin polymorphism and differential expression in adult human skeletal muscle. Comp. *Biochem. Physiol.* 106, 463-475, 1993

41. Staron, R.S., Leonardi, M.J., Karapondo, D.L., Malicky, E.S., Falkel, J.E., Hagerman, F.C., and Hikida, R.S. Strength and skeletal muscle adaptations in heavy-resistance-trained women after detraining and retraining. *J. Appl. Physiol.* 70, 631-640, 1991.

42. Staron, R.S., Malicky, E.S., Leonardi, M.J., Falkel, J.E., Hagerman, F.C., and, Dudley, G.A. Muscle hypertrophy and fast fiber type conversions in heavy resistance-trained woman. *Eur. J. Appl. Physiol.* 60, 71-79, 1990.

43. Tesch, P.A., and Karlsson, J. Muscle fiber types and size in trained and untrained muscles of elite athletes. *J. Appl. Physiol.* 59, 1716-1720, 1985.
44. Tesch, P.A., Komi, P.V. and, Häkkinen, K. Enzymatic adaptations consequent to long-term strength training. *Int. J. Sports Med.* 8, 66-69, 1987.
45. Thorstensson, A., Larsson, L., Tesch, P., and Karlsson, J. Muscle strength and fiber composition in athletes and sedentary men. *Med. Sci. Sports,* 9, 26-30, 1977.
46. Torok, D.J., Duey, W.J., Bassett, D.R., Howley, E.T., and Mancuso, P. Cardiovascular responses to exercise in sprinters and distance runners. *Med. Sci. Sports. Exerc.,* 27, 1050-1056, 1995.

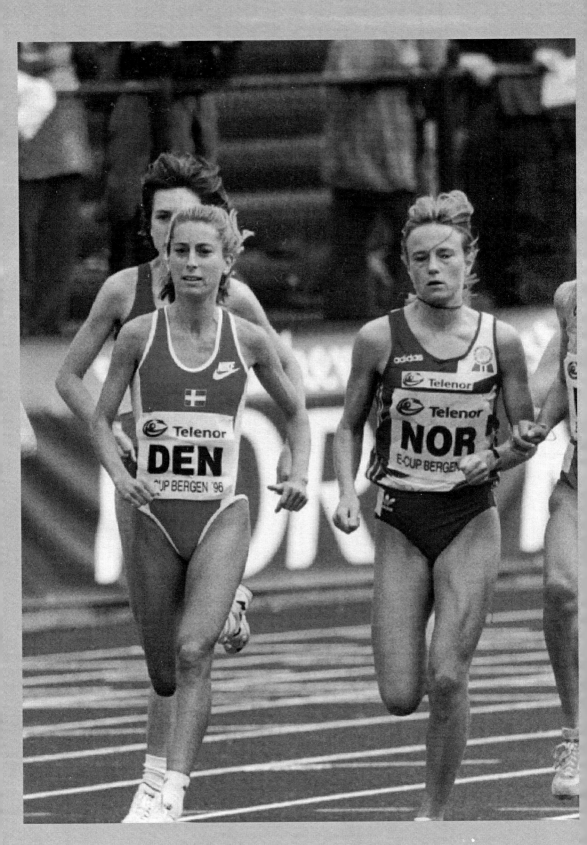

Physiological Factors Affecting Running Performance

Carlo Capelli & Pietro E. di Prampero

Synopsis

The present paper shows that by utilising a model based on the present physiological knowledge it is possible to predict fairly well theoretical best performance times and speeds in running provided that the following physiological variables of the subjects are known: maximal aerobic power (MAP), anaerobic lactic capacity (AnL), anaerobic alactic capacity (AnAl) and energy cost of running (Cr). Further manipulations of the model make it possible to quantify the impact of the same variables on performances. This showed that, among all the considered variables, the energy cost of running is the major determinant of the maximal speeds attained in running.

Introduction

The metabolic power required $(\dot{E}_r)$ to run a given distance d in the time t is set by the product of the energy cost of running (C_r) and the speed $(v = d \cdot t^{-1})$:

$$\dot{E}_r = C_r \cdot v = C_r \cdot d \cdot t^{-1} \qquad 1)$$

where C_r is the amount of metabolic energy spent to run over one unit of distance (15). Since C_r is constant or increases slightly with v, it necessarily follows that $\dot{E}_r$ is larger the smaller t. Thus, for any given distance and subject, the shortest time will be achieved when $\dot{E}_r$ is equal to the individual maximal metabolic power $(\dot{E}_{max})$. In turn, $\dot{E}_{max}$

is a known decreasing function of t: it depends on the subject's Maximal Aerobic Power (MAP) and on the maximal amount of energy derived from full utilisation of Anaerobic energy Stores (AnS) (16). So, if the relationship between C_r and v, together with the subject's MAP and AnS, are known, his or her Best Performance Time (BPT) over any given distance d can be obtained finding the time value which solves the equality $\dot{E}_{max}(t) = \dot{E}_r(t)$.

The paragraphs that follow will be devoted to illustrate that individual BPTs in track running can be predicted with satisfactory accuracy (16) utilising this approach. In addition, it will be shown that the same approach can be used also to quantify the role of the energy cost of running (C_r), of the Maximal Aerobic Power (MAP) and of the Anaerobic energy Stores (AnS) in determining BPTs in running.

Metabolic Power Requirement in Running

The overall energy cost per unit of distance of track running (C_r) from a stationary start on flat terrain is given by (16):

$$C_r = C_{r,na} + k' \cdot v^2 + (0.5\ v^2 \cdot d^{-1} \cdot \eta^{-1}) \qquad 2)$$

where: i) $C_{r,na}$ $(J \cdot m^{-1} \cdot kg^{-1})$ is the metabolic energy spent per unit of distance against non aerodynamic forces: in élite middle-distance runners it amounts, on the average, to 3.8 $J \cdot m^{-1} \cdot kg^{-1}$ (8); ii) k' is the proportionality constant between the energy cost against air drag and the square of the air speed: it amounts to ~ 0.40 $J \cdot s^2 \cdot m^{-3}$ per m² of body surface for a barometric pressure of 760 mmHg and an air temperature of 20°C (16); iii) the third term is the metabolic energy spent, over a unit of distance, to accelerate 1 kg body mass from zero to the final speed v: it is given by the kinetic energy per unit of distance and unit of body mass $(0.5\ v^2 \cdot d^{-1})$ divided by the overall efficiency of running (η) {eta}. As a first approximation, η {eta} can be assumed equal to 0.25 since, in the initial acceleration phase, no (or only very small) recovery of elastic energy can take place: hence the mechanical efficiency approaches that of the concentric muscular contraction (5). Substituting these values into Eq. 2, the overall metabolic energy spent per unit distance $(J \cdot m^{-1})$ for an élite runner of standard anthropometric characteristics (70 kg, 175 cm) can be described as:

$$C_r = 264.6 + 0.74\ v^2 + 140\ v^2 \cdot d_{tot}^{-1} \qquad 3)$$

This equation shows that, over the shorter distances and the faster speeds, the kinetic term (third term of Equation 3) is a substantial fraction of C_r. Indeed, for a 400 m run at speeds close to the absolute best performance (9.3 m•s^{-1}), the kinetic term amounts to about 7.5% of the overall energy cost. However, for longer distances and slower speeds, its weight becomes progressively smaller: at world record speeds it amounts to less than 1% in the 5000 m distance.

The overall metabolic power output necessary to run at speed v is given by the product of C_r and v (Equation 1). Once again, since in track running the distance of each competition is fixed and known, d t^{-1} can be substituted for v. Equation 3 becomes then:

$$\dot{E}_r = 264.6 \ d•t^{-1} + 0.74 \ d^3•t^{-3} + 140 \ d^2•t^3 \qquad 4)$$

The total metabolic power required $(\dot{E}_r)$ for covering 0.8 km in a time interval ranging from 80 to 120 s, for an élite athlete of 70 kg body mass and 175 cm height, as calculated from Equation 4, is shown in Figure 1A.

It goes without saying that equation 4 may yield $\dot{E}_r$ of any given subject over any given distance provided the individual value of $C_{r, na}$ is known, together with his/her anthropometric characteristics.

Maximal Metabolic Power

The maximal metabolic power $(\dot{E}_{max},$ kW) a given subject can sustain at a steady level throughout the effort is a decreasing function of the exhaustion time (t_e) (4, 16, 19); it can be appropriately described by:

$$\dot{E}_{max} = AnS•t_e^{-1} + [F•MAP - (F•MAP•\tau•(1 - e^{-k•\tau-1}))•t_e^{-1}] \qquad 5)$$

where:
i) AnS is the total metabolic energy obtained from complete utilisation of anaerobic sources, i.e. from anaerobic glycolysis and from net high energy phosphates splitting.
ii) MAP (Maximal Aerobic Power) is the equivalent in kW of the individual maximal oxygen consumption $(\dot{V}O_2\text{-max})$ measured above the oxygen consumption at rest;
iii) τ {tau} is the time constant with which MAP is attained at the onset of the effort;
iv) F is the fraction of MAP which can be sustained throughout the effort.

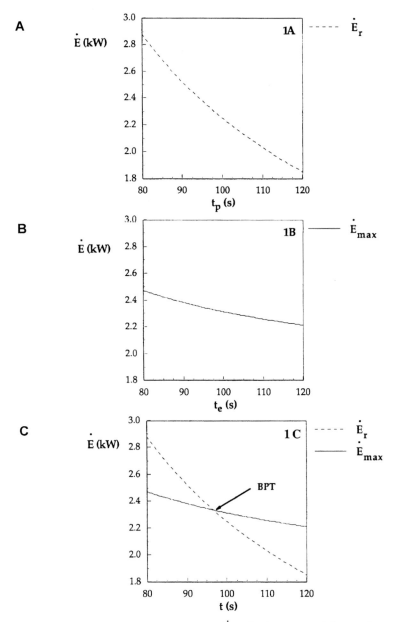

Figure 1. Metabolic power requirement ($\dot{E}_2$, kW) to run 0.8 km in the time indicated on the abscissa (A) and maximal available metabolic power ($\dot{E}_{max}$, kW) (B)
over the same time interval. Data were calculated for a hypothetical elite athlete
whose characteristics are as follows: body mass = 70 kg; gross $\dot{V}O_2$-max = 5.0 l ·
min^{-1}; Overall anaerobic capacity = 100 kJ. The time value at which the two
functions $\dot{E}_2$ and $\dot{E}_{max}$ cross yields the best performance time (BPT) of this
hypothetical athlete over this distance (C) see text for details.

The third term is due to the fact that $\dot{V}O_2$-max at the onset of exercise is not attained instantaneously, but with a time constant τ. Hence, the average aerobic power up to the time t_e is given by the quantity in square brackets, i.e. it is reduced below F•MAP by an amount equal to the O_2 deficit incurred to t_e (F•MAP•τ•$(1 - e^{-te\cdot\tau-1})$) divided by the time t_e itself. The first and third terms of equation 5 become progressively smaller with increasing t_e. So, equation 5 shows that, for long term exercise, the maximal sustainable metabolic power is essentially set by the subjects $\dot{V}O_2$-max and by the fraction of it which can be maintained throughout the effort. As the time of the exercise becomes shorter, the contribution of the anaerobic energy stores to the overall metabolic power becomes progressively greater. Indeed, with decreasing t_e, the first and third term of equation 5 become larger. Hence, not only does the anaerobic power becomes larger, but also the effective aerobic power is eroded by the increasing weight of the O_2 deficit.

Equation 5 shows that the time course of E_{max} can be described as a function of t_e for any given subject, provided the variables mentioned above are known. We will therefore proceed identifying the appropriate values of these variables for a „standard" élite athlete.

As mentioned above, AnS is the sum of the amount of energy derived from full exploitation of the anaerobic glycolytic pathway (anaerobic lactic capacity, AnL) plus that provided by maximal depletion of phosphocreatine and adenosine triphosphate (anaerobic alactic capacity, AnAl) in the working muscles. The former can be set equal to 1 kJ kg⁻¹ (14), and the latter increases with the duration of exhausting exercise with a time constant (τ_{al}) of 23.4 s to attain an asymptotic value of 0.42 kJ kg⁻¹ for exercises longer than 120 s (10). Hence, the overall anaerobic capacity of a 70 kg body mass subject (AnS, kJ) is described by:

$$AnS = (0.42\cdot(1-e^{-te/\tau al}) + 1.0)\cdot70 \tag{6}$$

Assuming a gross $\dot{V}O_2$-max of 5.0 l min⁻¹, a value typical for élite athletes (15), and an oxygen consumption at rest of 3.5 ml O_2 min⁻¹ kg⁻¹, the maximal metabolic power (MAP) turns out to be 1.66 kW for a subject of 70 kg.

The time constant of the simple exponential function describing the increase of $\dot{V}O_2$ at muscular level at the onset of the maximal exercise (τ), as measured by means of ³¹P nuclear magnetic resonance spectroscopy (1), is on the order of 24 s. So, for the values of MAP and of

AnS mentioned above, the weight of the third term of equation 5 decreases with increasing t_e from about 20% of $\dot{E}_{max}$ for $t_e = 40$ s to less than 4% for $t_e = 10$ minutes.

The fraction of MAP sustainable throughout the effort (F) depends on the duration of the exercise. For t_e longer than 7 minutes, it can be assumed to decrease linearly with the logarithm of t_e (13). Accordingly, F in Eq. 5 takes the following values:

$$F \begin{cases} = 1.00; & \text{for } 45 \text{ s} < t_e < 420 \text{ s} \\ = 1 - 0.0568 \ln (t_e/420); & \text{for } > 420 \text{ s} \end{cases} \qquad 7)$$

The values reported above allowed us to calculate the maximal available metabolic power $(\dot{E}_{max})$ for a hypothetical élite athlete; it is represented in Figure 1B as a function of t_e over the same time range as in Figure 1A.

It also goes without saying that the knowledge of the individual values of MAP and AnS, together with the subject's anthropometric features, would allow us to describe $\dot{E}_{max}$ as function of t_e in any given individual.

Best Performance Times

Figure 1C shows that for a certain range of t values, $\dot{E}_{max}$ is below the function describing the metabolic power requirement $(\dot{E}_r)$. These times will therefore be unattainable by this subject. For longer t values, $\dot{E}_{max}$ is above $\dot{E}_r$. Therefore, this hypothetical athlete could have covered the distance at stake in a shorter time. It seems therefore reasonable to assume that the theoretical best time of performance (t_{theor}) is given by the abscissa at which the two functions cross. In practice, the time value solving the equalities $\dot{E}_{max}(t_e) = \dot{E}_r(t)$; i.e. t_{theor}, can be obtained graphically, as in Figure 1C, or by means of a computerised iterative procedure on the basis of the values of AnS, MAP and C_r and assuming a value of τ.

The approach described above was tested in a group of 16 male and female runners of intermediate level competing in middle distance running (age: 18.2 ± 2.7 yrs; body mass: 60.0 ± 8.7 kg; height: 173.8 ± 7.4 cm; $\dot{V}O_2$-max: 55.2 ± 7.6 ml min^{-1} kg^{-1}) in whom steady-state oxygen consumption $(\dot{V}O_2$, ml min^{-1} kg$^{-1})$ and blood lactate concentration

($[La]_b$, mM) were determined during constant speed track running (speed range: 3.66–6.00 m s^{-1}) (16). Energy cost of running was calculated from the ratio of $\dot{V}O_2$ above resting to speed and expressed in joules per kilogram of body mass per meter assuming an energetic equivalent of 20.9 J per ml O_2 (16). When $[La]_b$ at the end of the run exceeded 2.0 mM, the energy cost was corrected for the amount of metabolic energy derived from glycolysis. This was accomplished assuming that the net increase of one mmol/l of lactate ($\nabla[La]_b$) above the value prevailing before the trial is equal to 60 J per mM per kilogram of body mass (3 ml O_2 kg^{-1} mM^{-1}) (15) in terms of metabolic energy yield. The energy cost of running turned out to be essentially independent of the speed and amounted, on the average, to 3.72±0.24 J m^{-1} kg^{-1}.

Since in this study the energy cost was determined during track running, it included the amount of energy spent per meter against air drag. Hence, Equation 2 reduced to:

$$C_r = C + (0.5 \ v^2 \cdot d^{-1} \cdot \eta^{-1})$$

where C corresponded to the individual energy cost of running assessed on the track as described above. This made it possible to calculate $\dot{E}_r$ of each subject over a set of running distances on which the subjects had been competing in the same season and over time ranges including, for each subject and distance, his/her BPT.

$\dot{E}_{max}$ of each subject was obtained inserting the individual value of $\dot{V}O_2$-max in Equation 5, together with the appropriate values of AnS. This last was assumed to amount to 1.42 kJ per kilogram of body mass in a 25-yrs old male athlete and to be smaller in younger subjects (83% of the above at 16 yrs and 94% at 19 yrs) (6).

So, the individual $\dot{E}_r$ and $\dot{E}_{max}$ functions could be described analytically for each subject and distance as shown above (see Figure 1C), thus allowing us to calculate the theoretical BPTs and to compare them with the actual seasonal BPTs over the very same distances.
The same set of calculations was then applied to a similar set of data reported by Lacour et al. (8) for French elite athletes.

For both groups of subjects theoretical and actual BPTs are plotted against each other in Figure 2 and theoretical and actual best performance speeds in Figure 3. In all cases, the experimental relationships between theoretical and actual values showed rather high determination coefficients and were rather close to the identity line, thus showing that the model could predict actual performances fairly well. This is

73

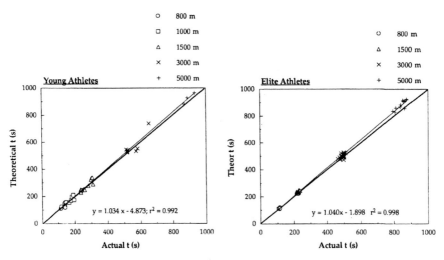

Figure 2. Theoretical best performance times are plotted as a function of actual seasonal records for young runners (left diagram) and for French élite athletes (from 8, right diagram).

also shown in Figure 4 where the differences of the logarithms of the actual and theoretical BPTs are plotted as a function of the logarithm of their mean: the differences lay generally between the values of the overall mean of the differences plus or minus two standard deviations, thus confirming the satisfactory precision of the prediction.

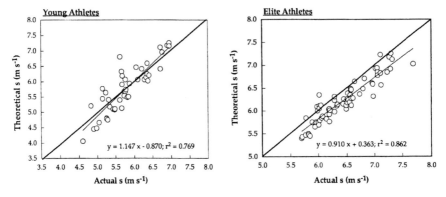

Figure 3. Theoretical best performance speeds are plotted as a function of the actual seasonal records for young runners (left diagram) and for French élite athletes (from 8, right diagram).

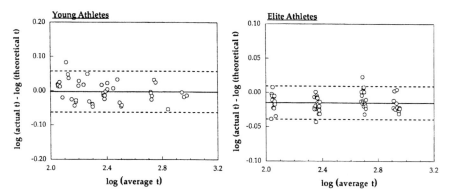

Figure 4. Differences between natural logarithms of actual and theoretical best performance time as a function of the logarithm of the corresponding average. The differences lay, in almost all the cases, between the averages (thick continuous lines) plus or minus one standard deviation (dotted lines). Left panel: young athletes; right panel: French élite athletes.

In summary, the proposed model allowed us to predict with fairly good accuracy best performance times in different groups of runners over distances from 0.8 to 5.0 km. A possible source of error was probably due to the fact that the time constant t and the maximal capacity of the anaerobic energy sources (AnS) were assumed averages rather than individual values. Hence, better predictions can be expected utilising actual individual data of t and AnS.

This aspect of the model will not be discussed further, the reader being referred to previous published works (4, 16). The paragraphs that follow will be devoted to show that the model described above makes it possible to quantify the weight of its physiological inputs in determining best running performances. Indeed we think that the main utility of this approach consists in allowing the trainer to make this type of evaluation rather than in the possibility, that it also offers, to predict individual BPT, in which case even a 5 percent error (as observed on the average) would make the model of little practical use.

Physiological Factors Affecting Running Performance

The procedure illustrated above can be utilised to calculate to what extent the physiological inputs, namely MAP, AnL, AnAl and C, affect performance. To this aim, best performance times in running is calculated over various distances applying initial, pre-defined values for MAP, C, AnL and AnAl. The procedure is then repeated modifying one variable at a time by discrete and pre-defined intervals above and below the initial control value, i.e. the value utilised in the first run of the simulation. This procedure, if applied for each variable and distances, will bring about calculated percent increases (or decreases) of best performance times.

The simulation illustrated above will now be applied to a standard élite athlete running over the distance of 1.5 km from a stationary start. The four input variables will be varied by 2.5% steps over an interval ranging from 90 to 100% of the following control values: MAP, C_r, AnL and AnAL. For the overall energy cost of running, the 2.5% changes will be applied to its non aerodynamic fraction ($C_{r,\,na}$ in equation 2). The results obtained when changing only MAP are reported in Figure 5. The nine thin curves describe $\dot{E}_{max}$ as a function of t_e. The abscissa values at which these nine curves cross the dashed thick $\dot{E}_{r,\,tot}$ function form the set of the best performance times obtained when MAP was changed from 90 to 110% of the initial values, while the other three variables remained constant. Obviously enough, three other sets of

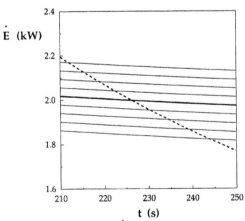

Figure 5. Metabolic power requirement $\dot{E}_2$ (dashed thick line) to run 1.5 km in the time indicated on the abscissa. Maximal available metabolic power max is also indicated (continuous thick curve) on the same time axis. Data apply to an élite athlete whose characteristics are as follows: body mass = 70 kg; gross VO_2-max = 5.0 l•min⁻¹; Overall anaerobic capacity = 100 kJ. Thin curves correspond to the maximal metabolic power available when MAP above the value at rest is smaller or larger than 1.66 kW. Best performance times becomes shorter as MAP increases from 90% to 110% of 1.66 kW. See text for details.

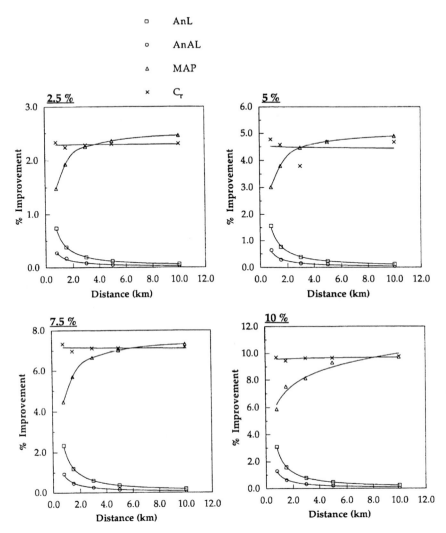

Figure 6. Percent improvement of the initial best performance time in running as a function of the distance when the four indicated variables of the model (AnL; AnAl; MAP; Cr) are changed by 2.5, 5, 7.5 and 10%.

BPTs are obtained when the other three variables (AnL, AnAl and C_r) are changed as described.

The percent improvements of the initial best performance times in running are summarised in Figure 6 as a function of the distance covered (d, km) and for 2.5, 5.0, 7.5 and 10.0% changes of the four variables. Each curve describes the results obtained when only the indicated variable was modified. Each curve was drawn by eye interpolating the data only for the sake of description. These diagrams give an immediate representation of the weight of each of the four variables in determining the performance in running. For instance, the improvement achieved by modifying either the maximal aerobic power or the overall anaerobic capacity depends on the distance (and hence on the time of performance). On the contrary, the improvement achieved by modifying only C_r remains essentially constant regardless of the distance (and time) indicating that the improvements brought about by changes of C_r are hardly affected by the metabolic power output.

The results of the foregoing analysis are summarised further in Figure 7, where the improvement in performance due to a 5.0% change (decrease) of C_r expressed as a fraction of the overall improvement obtained when all the four variables determining performance (C_r, decrease; MAP, AnL, AnAl, increase) are changed, each by the same amount (5.0%), is plotted as a function of the time of performance. The diagram shows that the extent of improvement achieved by decreasing C_r alone is comparable to that attained by increasing simultaneously MAP, AnAl and AnL by the same percentage. Moreover, this is affected only to a little extent by the time of performance.

Figures 6 and 7 show unambiguously that the single variable whose changes most effectively influence performance is C_r. However, for practical purposes, it is often convenient to know the percent change

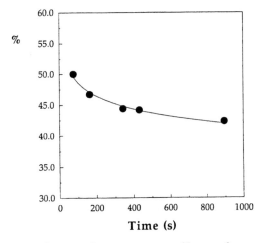

Figure 7. The ratio (%) between the improvement of best performance time brought about by 5% changes of Cr only to that obtained by changing all four variables by the same amount is plotted as function of the time in running.

of performance brought about by any given change(s) by any prede-termined amount(s) of all four variables at stake. Obviously enough, these calculations can be easily done algebraically. For convenience, an example of such an approach is reported for the distances of 1.5, 3.0 and 10 km in Figure 8 where the linear functions represent the percent increase, or decrease, of the best performance time over the appropriate distance when the variable at stake is changed by the amount indicated on the abscissa. The point upon which all lines pivot corresponds to the theoretical best time of performance when all varia-bles are set at their initial control value. In Figure 8, the relationships between the percent increase or decrease of the performance time and the percent change of the independent variable were assumed to be linear. However, since neither $\dot{E}_r$ nor $\dot{E}_{max}$ are linear functions of the performance time, the above assumption is an obvious oversimpli-fication. Nevertheless, within the range of the independent variable reported in Figure 8, these relationships can be approximated by li-near regressions whose slopes are reported in Table 1 (mean $r^2 = 0.997 \pm 0.0019$, range: 1.000–0.993).The advantage of this oversimplification is that linear effects can be easily added. For instance, the effects deriving from a 5.0% increase of MAP and from a 3.0% increase of AnL can be added to yield the overall percent decrease of the theoretical best time of performance. Table 1 makes it possible to apply this type of theoretical analysis to all the running distances considered.

Table 1. Percent decrease or increase of theoretical best times of performance obtained changing by one percent MAP, AnAl, AnL and C in running. Time values in seconds indicate best times of performance obtained utilising the initial values of MAP, AnAl, AnL and C representing the physiological characteristics of a hypothetical élite athlete.

Distance m	Time t sec	t / MAP, %	t / AnAl, %	t / Anl, %	t / C, %
400	39.5	-0.288	-0.202	-0.613	0.027
800	109.7	-0.622	-0.128	-0.310	0.933
1500	237.5	-0.784	-0.065	-0.158	0.886
3000	519	-0.897	-0.034	-0.080	0.902
5000	919.2	-0.897	-0.020	-0.048	0.901
10000	1963.4	-0.997	-0.010	-0.024	0.907

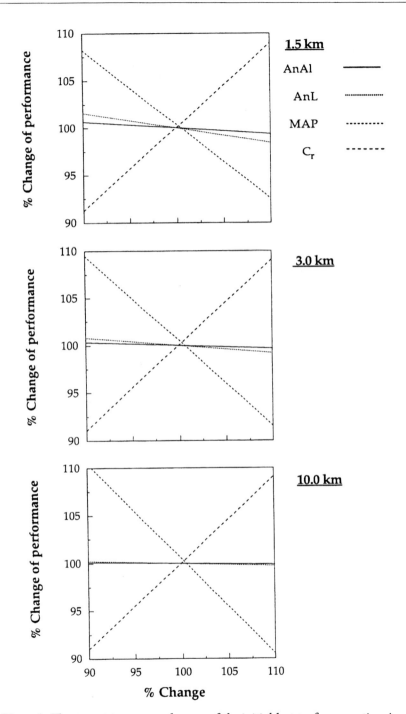

Figure 8. The percent increase or decrease of the initial best performance time is plotted as a function of the percent change of MAP, AnAl, AnL or overall Cr for the three indicated distances.

General Discussion

The results of the above analysis depend on several assumptions, particularly as far as the form of the equations is concerned. Hence, the few paragraphs that follow will be devoted to discuss the dependence of the results on the assumptions made.

Equations similar to that yielding $\dot{E}_{max}$ as function of t_e (Equation 5) have been applied in the past to calculate theoretical best performance times in runners (see above and in reference 4) and in élite cyclists over several distances (4, 16). Theoretical and actual times agreed well, and all assumptions on which Equation 5 is based have been extensively discussed in the quoted papers to which the reader is referred. Equation 5 has been also recently utilised to estimate the energy cost of swimming (3) and running (7) at supramaximal speeds. Hence, we are fairly confident that the physiological premises on which Equation 5 is based are sufficiently solid to allow us to obtain an accurate description of the individual $\dot{E}_{max}$ as a function of t_e.

Maximal aerobic power has been reported to be significantly larger after high intensity training both in moderately active subjects and in élite athletes. For instance, $\dot{V}O_2$-max increased by 13% after six weeks of high-intensity intermittent exercise in a group of 7 physical education students (18) and it rose significantly from winter to the competitive mid-year season (+4.5%) in a group of well-trained high level track runners (17). Also anaerobic capacity can be substantially increased by high intensity raining. This was shown to occur, for instance, in moderately active, young male subjects in whom anaerobic capacity rose by 28% at the end of 6 weeks of intense, intermittent cycle ergometric exercise and in sprint – trained subjects whose anaerobic capacity was 10% larger at the end of six weeks of high intensity running training (11). Therefore, the percent changes imposed to MAP and to anaerobic capacities in the simulations reported above (see Figure 6) reproduce fairly well those brought about by the training or detraining in élite athletes.

At variance with $\dot{V}O_2$-max and anaerobic capacity, there is far from a consensus as to the effects of training on running economy (2, 9), even though cross-sectional studies have often revealed that C_r is lower in long-distance runners and in adult subjects than in sprint runners and in children (12). Moreover C_r seems to be identical between similarly trained male and female athletes (2). More recently, a retrospective analysis of seven publications spanning a period of twenty years re-examined the differences in the cost of running among three groups of runners who were stratified according to the different performance level (12). The study revealed that élite runners were more economical than the less talented ones and that, on the average, trained subjects had a better running economy than untrained controls. However, within-group variability was high in all the groups and there was also a substantial overlap of minimum, mean and maximal value of running economy over the categories. Hence, it is not clear whether long distance training does improve running economy or whether long distance runners naturally select endurance events because of their innate economy which can be maximally exploited over the longest distances rather than during sprint events. In spite of these uncertainties, the analysis presented in this paper suggests that C_r should be always assessed in runners.

Summary

In conclusion, the analysis illustrated in the present paper showed that a theoretical model based on present physiological knowledge can predict fairly well theoretical best performance times and speeds in running, provided some physiological variables (C_r, MAP, AnL and AnAl) of the subjects are known. In addition, further manipulations of the same theoretical model make it possible to quantify the impact of the same physiological variables on performances. The analysis showed that, among the considered variables, C_r turned out to be the major determinant of the maximal speeds attained in running when all the distances were considered. We think that the approach illustrated here above might be fruitfully extended to animal physiology so as to investigate the physiological determinants of maximal speeds in several forms of animal locomotion.

References

1. Binzoni, T, Ferretti, G., Shenker, K. et al Phosphocreatine hydrolysis by 31P - NMR at the onset of constant---load exercise in humans. *J. Appl. Physiol.* 73, 1644--1649, 1992.

2. Bourdin, M., Pastene, J., Germain, M. et al Influence of training, sex, age and body mass on the energy cost of running. *Eur. J. Appl. Physiol.* 66, 439-444 1993.

3. Capelli, C, Pendergast, D. R. and Termin, B. Energetics of swimming at maximal speeds. *Eur. J. Appl. Physiol.* 78, 385-393 1998.

4. Capelli, C., Schena, F., Zamparo, P. et al Energetics of best performances in track cycling. *Med Sci Sports Exerc.* 30: 614-624, 1998.

5. Cavagna, G., Komarek, L. and Mazzoleni, S. The mechanics of sprint running. *J. Physiol (London)* 217, 709-721, 1971.

6. Cerretelli, P., Aghemo, P. and Rovelli, E. Aspetti fisiologici dell'adolescente in relazione alla pratica dell'esercizio fisico. *Med. Sport Turin* 21: 731-734, 1968.

7. Hautier, C.A., Wouassi, D., Arsac, L.M. et al Relationships between postcompetition blood lactate concentration and average runing velocity over 100---m and 200---m races. *Eur. J. Appl. Physiol.* 68, 508-513, 1994.

8. Lacour, J.R., Padilla-Magunacelaya, S., Barthélémy, J. C. et al The energetics of middle---distance running. *Eur. J. Appl. Physiol.* 60, 38-43, 1990.

9. Lake, M. J. and Cavanagh, P. R. Six weeks of training does not change running mechanics or improve running economy. *Med. Sci. Sports Exerc.* 28, 860-869, 1996.

10. Medbø, J. I. and Tabata, I. Anaerobic energy release in working muscle during 30 s to 3 min of exhausting bicycling. *J. Appl. Physiol.* 75, 1654-1660, 1993.

11. Medbø, J.I. and Burgers, S. Effect of training on the anaerobic capacity. *Med. Sci. Sports Exerc.* 22: 501-507, 1990.

12. Morgan, D.W., Brannsford, D.R., Costill, D.L., et al Variation in the aerobic demand of running among trained and untrained subjects. Med. Sci. Sports Exerc. 27, 404-409, 1995.

13. Péronnet, F. and Thibault, G. Mathematical analysis of running performance and world running records. *J. Appl. Physiol.* 67, 453-465, 1989.

14. Prampero di, P. E. Energetics of muscular exercise. *Rev. Physiol. Biochem. Pharmacol.* 89, 143-222, 1981.

15. Prampero di, P.E. The energy cost of human locomotion on land and in water. *Int. J. Sports Med.* 7, 55-72, 1986.

16. Prampero di, P.E., Capelli, C., Pagliaro, P. et al Energetics of best performances in middle-distance running. *J. Appl. Physiol.* 74, 2318-2324, 1993.

17. Svedenhag, J. and Sjödin, B. Physical characteristics of elite male runners in and off-season. *Can. J. Appl. Sport Sci.* 10, 127-133, 1985.

18. Tabata, I., Nishimura, K., Kouzaki, M. et al Effects of moderate---intensity endurance and high---intensity intermittent training on anaerobic capacity and VO_2-max. *J. Appl. Physiol.* 28, 1327-1330, 1996.

19. Wilkie, D. R. Equations describing power input by humans as a function of duration of exercise; In *Exercise Bioenergetics and Gas Exchange,* P. Cerretelli and B. J. Whipp eds, Elsevier, Amsterdam, The Netherlands, pp 75-80, 1980.

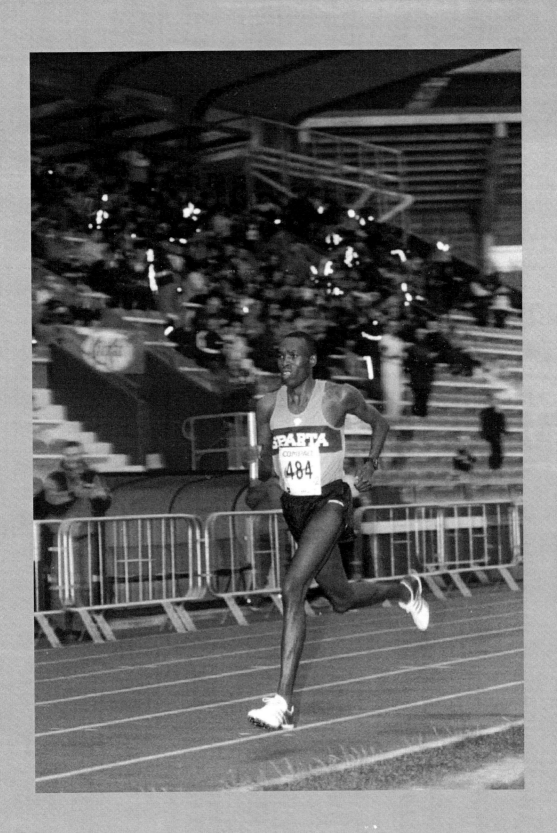

Running Economy

Jan Svedenhag

Synopsis

Running economy is one important factor determining running capacity in endurance events, but it should be expressed in a proper way, preferably in $ml \cdot kg^{0.75} \cdot min^{-1}$. Given test conditions are well controlled, running economy seems to be a quite robust measure. It may, however, change within a single exercise bout or with long-term training. Of the many factors that may determine running economy, the ability to store/use elastic energy in the running musculature and tendons may be especially important.

Introduction

The increased interest during the last decades in endurance training and especially long-distance running has created unique opportunities for more thorough studies on the physiology of racing performances in endurance events. This has led to a better understanding of the factors determining endurance capacity. One such important factor is the steady-state submaximal oxygen uptake at given running velocities, i.e. the running economy.

In the present chapter, different aspects of running economy will be presented. But before we turn to discuss these matters any further, let me first give a background on how oxygen uptake during running is thought to be related to performance in human subjects.

Oxygen uptake related to endurance running performance

Maximal oxygen uptake

Since the 1930s it has been known that the maximal oxygen uptake ($\dot{V}O_2$-max) is exceptionally high in elite endurance event athletes. These high values are thought to be due to a combination of training effort and natural endowment. Early studies of elite runners (3, 60) measured values of up to 81.5 ml•kg^{-1}•min^{-1} in champion athletes. This is comparable to the $\dot{V}O_2$-max observed in elite runners of today; for example mean for a 5000-10000 m group of Swedish elite runners 78.7 ml•kg^{-1}•min^{-1} (66). Thus, improvements in competitive results for middle and long distances seen over the last 50 years cannot be ascribed to a higher $\dot{V}O_2$-max of today's elite runners. Although evidently important, the maximal oxygen uptake is only one of the factors that determines success in middle- and long-distance events. This is illustrated by the large variation in performance between marathon runners of equal $\dot{V}O_2$-max and vice versa (see 61).

Running economy

Since the early 1970s, there has been growing interest in how to utilise best the maximal aerobic capacity in endurance events. During running, the submaximal oxygen uptake of an individual is directly and linearly related to his/her running velocity. However, at a given running speed, the submaximal oxygen requirement (in ml•kg^{-1}•min^{-1}) may vary considerably between subjects (18, 66). The lower the $\dot{V}O_2$-submax at a given running speed the better the running economy. In elite distance runners with a relatively narrow range in $\dot{V}O_2$-max, the running economy at different speeds has been found to be significantly correlated (r = 0.79-0.83) with performance at a 10-km race (16). A low $\dot{V}O_2$-submax (i.e. good running economy) is thus truly beneficial. There is also a surprisingly wide (up to 20%) individual variation in running economy (ml•kg^{-1}•min^{-1}) at 15 km•h^{-1} between marathon runners of the good or elite level (61). In contrast, the differences may be small or non-existent when groups of elite runners from different distances are compared (66). Furthermore, in a heterogeneous material, there may be a relatively poor correlation between the $\dot{V}O_2$-submax during running and endurance performance at a specific distance, e.g. r = -0.55 in a marathon with a large variation in performance (61). Also, within a narrower performance range (2:30-3:00 Marathon) no significant correlation between running economy and performance (r = 0.25, n = 16; 24) seems to be typical.

It has been recognised that both $\dot{V}O_2$-max and running economy has to be taken into account for the prediction of running performance (52, 66). A given performance at an endurance event, such as running, can also be attained in different ways. Two kinds of elite runners with different physiological characteristics can be distinguished. One category of runners is characterised by a high maximal oxygen uptake ($\dot{V}O_2$-max) but a relatively poor running economy. The second category of runners has an excellent running economy, but a relatively low $\dot{V}O_2$-max. In many cases the overall result of these differences is a fairly even performance level (53, 66). Both the accomplished training and various natural abilities may contribute to these differences in running economy (see below) and in $\dot{V}O_2$-max. Only an outstanding runner may have good or excellent values in both running economy and $\dot{V}O_2$-max.

Running economy related to $\dot{V}O_2$-max

In order to help in accounting for individual differences in running economy and $\dot{V}O_2$-max in relation to performance, the fractional utilisation of $\dot{V}O_2$-max when running at a specific speed (e.g. 15 km•h^{-1} or 18 km•h^{-1}) can be calculated. The % $\dot{V}O_2$-max value calculated in this way has been found to be significantly correlated to performance at various long distances. This value can be regarded as an *aerobic running capacity* of a runner. For instance, in the heterogeneous group of marathon runners mentioned above (61), the relationship between fractional utilisation of $\dot{V}O_2$ max at a submaximal speed of 15 km•h^{-1} and performance was very good (r = -0.94, n=35). This is because the % $\dot{V}O_2$-max value expresses the combined effects of $\dot{V}O_2$-max and of running economy, both of which may be separately related to performance.

In recent years, another way of expressing the combined effect of running economy and $\dot{V}O_2$-max has gained popularity. This refers to the so called predicted velocity at $\dot{V}O_2$-max ($v\dot{V}O_2$-max; 43). In this approach the linear relationship between running speed and submaximal oxygen utilisation of an individual is extrapolated up to his/her $\dot{V}O_2$-max value and the running velocity at which this would be attained is employed. If the running economy extrapolation can be accepted, this may be the preferred way of expression, particularly for middle-distance runners with high racing velocities.

Methodological considerations

Variability

During running at submaximal velocities, steady-state energy condition is thought to be attained in about 3 min (42). Thus, for appropriate measurements to be done, each submaximal level should be at least 4 min long. With this in mind, several authors have investigated the intra-individual variation in $\dot{V}O_2$-submax during running on the treadmill. Most studies have yielded low coefficients of variation of 1.3 - 4.6% (12, 45, 57, 69, 76) under conditions in which time of day, training activity, footwear and treadmill accommodation were controlled to some extent. Of this error in running economy in repeated measurements, biological variation is thought to play a large role (57). Furthermore, measurements of running economy seem to be quite robust in that 30 min maximal runs in moderately to well-trained runners did not produce any significant changes in running economy when tested 1, 2 and 4 days after the run (44, 49).

Scaling factors

Background
When comparing biologic functions between animals or humans of different sizes, or within individuals with changing body masses, a strictly dimensional thinking is often enlightening. In these comparisons static and dynamic functions are expressed as being proportional to multiples of the linear dimension (L). In this way, the effect of body

dimensions on several performance and/or capacity measures can be calculated (4). For example, the oxygen uptake ($\dot{V}O_2$, $l\cdot min^{-1}$) has been shown to be proportional to L^2. Therefore, $\dot{V}O_2$ ($l\cdot min^{-1}$) should be proportional to the body mass raised to the 2/3 power (see also 65) and not as most commonly done to body mass in the first power.

In studying the relationship between resting as well as maximal oxygen uptake and body mass in mammals (from the mouse or dwarf mangoose to the elephant or eland), power values of 0.73 - 0.79 have been found (for references see 65). Obviously this differs considerably from body mass to the 1.0 power but also, albeit less, from the 2/3 power of body mass from a strictly dimensional aspect as outlined above. However, based on calculated limitations imposed by elastic components of biological material, metabolic rates have been suggested to be proportional to the 3/4 power of the body mass (40). Another proposed explanation is related to the fact that larger mammals have a greater proportion of proximal leg muscle mass in relation to their body mass (5, 51). In line with this, it has been hypothesised that an individual who possesses a relatively greater amount of his/her body mass in the extremities would thereby have to perform a relatively greater amount of work moving body segments during running than an individual with relatively lesser amount of body mass in the legs (50). This latter hypothesis has also been supported by several loading studies (see 42).

Regarding power values in human studies, von Döbeln (25) found that $\dot{V}O_2$-max was related to fat-free body mass raised to the power of 0.71 in a mixed population (both sexes). From calculations based on a large series of tests on adult humans, Bergh et al. (9) found that submaximal and maximal $\dot{V}O_2$ attained during running were related to the body mass raised to the powers of 0.76 and 0.71, respectively, and suggested that $\dot{V}O_2$ during running is better related to $kg^{2/3}$ or $kg^{3/4}$ than to kg^1. Furthermore, Sjödin & Svedenhag (62) suggested that changes in running economy and $\dot{V}O_2$-max ($ml\cdot kg^{-1}\cdot min^{-1}$) in adolescent boys during growth may be largely due to an overestimation of the $\dot{V}O_2$ dependence on body mass during running and favoured oxygen uptake being expressed per $kg^{3/4}$. Earlier as well as recent reports of an inverse relationship between body mass and $\dot{V}O_2$-submax or $\dot{V}O_2$-max during running (11, 31, 53, 56, 75) provide further support to this conception. For example, Bourdin et al (11) found correlation coefficients of $r = -0.47 - -0.76$ between energy cost of running

Table 1. Running economy ($\dot{V}O_2$-18) and aerobic running capacity ($\dot{V}O_2$-18/$\dot{V}O_2$-max) at 18 km·h^{-1} (= 5.0 m·s^{-1}) together with maximal oxygen uptake ($\dot{V}O_2$-max) in two elite runners with different body mass. The interpretation of the running economy and $\dot{V}O_2$-max results are clearly altered if related to kg$^{-0.75}$ instead of kg^{-1}. For further explanation see text.

	Body mass (kg)	$\dot{V}O_2$-18/$\dot{V}O_2$-max (%)	$\dot{V}O_2$-18 (ml·kg^{-1}·min^{-1})	$\dot{V}O_2$-18 (ml·kg$^{-0.75}$·min^{-1})	$\dot{V}O_2$-max (ml·kg^{-1}·min^{-1})	$\dot{V}O_2$-max (ml·kg$^{-0.75}$·min^{-1})
Runner A	80	75	55.5	166	74.0	221
Runner B	50	75	61.5	164	82.0	218

and body mass in different groups. Thus, several lines of evidence suggest that oxygen uptake determined during submaximal or maximal treadmill running should be related to kg$^{0.75}$ rather than to kg^{-1}.

Implications for the evaluation of the athlete

In Table 1, the effect of body-mass-normalisation on running economy and $\dot{V}O_2$-max in two athletes of clearly differing body masses are exemplified. The two elite runners have equal total aerobic running capacity (see above) and similar racing performance levels. Judged from their $\dot{V}O_2$-submax values (ml·kg^{-1}·min^{-1}) at 18 km·h^{-1} ($\dot{V}O_2$-18), the lighter runner B is having a clearly higher $\dot{V}O_2$-18 and thus would be regarded as having a worse running economy than the heavier runner A (Table 1). In evaluating the athletes' test results, runner B would be advised accordingly to concentrate more on training that improves the running economy. However, when expressed as ml·kg$^{-0.75}$·min^{-1}, the running economy ($\dot{V}O_2$-max- 18) of these two runners were similar, if anything, with runner B having a better value.

A reverse pattern is seen for $\dot{V}O_2$-max (Table 1). Here the heavier runner A is having a clearly lesser value when expressed as ml·kg^{-1}·min^{-1}; he would accordingly be advised to concentrate more on training that may improve the aerobic power. However, when expressed as ml•kg$^{-0.75}$•min^{-1}, the $\dot{V}O_2$-max of these two runners were similar, if anything, with runner A having a better value. Hence, the examples illustrate well how important it is to express properly the oxygen uptake during running for correct evaluation of athletes and other test subjects. Also, when comparing groups of individuals with differing body weights or in longitudinal studies of subjects with changing body masses is this new and "body-mass-modified" approach to running economy and $\dot{V}O_2$-max of great importance.

With this improved expression of running economy and $\dot{V}O_2$-max, new reference values must be created. Therefore, to put such new figures in proper context, Svedenhag & Sjödin (69) reported values for running economy and $\dot{V}O_2$-max (ml•kg$^{-0.75}$•min^{-1}) in two groups of elite male distance runners (Table 2). In this study, the oxygen uptake per unit distance run (i.e. the oxygen cost of running) was also calculated and the mean value was found to be 0.544 l•kg$^{-0.75}$•km^{-1}. This is in agreement with Morgan et al (48) as they reported the mean value in three groups of male runners (elite, sub-elite and good runners) to range from 0.514 to 0.552 l•kg$^{-0.75}$•km^{-1}.

Table 2. $\dot{V}O_2$-submax and $\dot{V}O_2$-max in ml•kg$^{-0.75}$•min^{-1} in two groups of elite runners

	Middle-distance runners	Long-distance runners
$\dot{V}O_2$-15	138 (129-148)	129 (116-139)
$\dot{V}O_2$-18	169 (158-179)	164 (151-174)
$\dot{V}O_2$-max	202 (184-216)	214 (193-232)

Factors related to running economy

Distance

In well-trained runners, the oxygen cost of running (C; in l•kg^{-1}•km^{-1} or ml•kg^{-1}•m^{-1}) has earlier been reported to be constant in the 60-95% $\dot{V}O_2$-max range (31, 55). However, when going from 15 to 18 km•h^{-1}

in elite runners (4 min at each velocity), Svedenhag & Sjödin (69) found small but significant increases in oxygen cost of running ($l \cdot kg^{-0.75} \cdot km^{-1}$) in both elite middle- (MD) and long-distance (LD) runners (MD: +2.2%, when going from 68 to 84% $\dot{V}O_2$-max; LD: +6.0%, from 60 to 77% $\dot{V}O_2$-max). The significantly greater difference in the long-distance runners may at least partly be an adaptation to great volumes of distance training in these runners resulting in a better running economy at slow speeds. The middle-distance runners may then be somewhat more economical than long-distance runners at higher running velocities, a finding also reported by Daniels & Daniels (22) when comparing running economy (in $ml \cdot kg^{-1} \cdot min^{-1}$, 6 min at each velocity) of 800/ 1500 m runners (male and female) to marathon runners of similar body masses. On the other hand, when running at high velocities with the submaximal oxygen uptake being close to $\dot{V}O_2$-max, the $\dot{V}O_2$ obtained may slightly underestimate total energy demand. This is based on studies using one-legged knee-extensor exercise, in which the anaerobic energy contribution at demanding submaximal exercise may be up to 10% above that produced by aerobic metabolism (8).

Training & tapering

Morgan et al. (48) analysed the oxygen cost of running (both as $ml \cdot kg^{-1} \cdot km^{-1}$ and as $ml \cdot kg^{-0.75} \cdot km^{-1}$) in three groups of trained distance runners (elite, sub-elite and good runners, n= 16-41) and in a group of untrained subjects (n=10). They concluded that 1) trained subjects are more economical than untrained subjects, 2) elite runners display better running economy compared to less talented counterparts, and that 3) economical and uneconomical runners can be found in all performance categories. Qualitatively, this is very much in line with findings earlier presented by Sjödin & Svedenhag (61) in different groups of marathon runners (elite, good and slow runners; see also above).

The question then arises if these differences in running economy are due just to effects of the performed training per se or to different inherent capacities in different individuals followed by a selection process (of those that continue being devoted). Or it may be a combination of the two possibilities.

A few studies have looked into this in adult subjects. From the results, it would seem that running economy is not readily trainable. Thus, studies on recreational and collegiate runners (21, 73) as well as on untrained volunteers (35) have not found any change in running economy after 6-8 weeks of running training (long-distance running and for the former two studies also interval training). On the other hand, a 14 week program of once a week anaerobic threshold training (20 min at 4 mmol•l^{-1} of blood lactate) added to the normal training program has been shown to increase the anaerobic threshold in 8 competitive middle- and long-distance runners, an effect which was partially mediated by an improvement in running economy (3%; 63). This is compatible with the improved running economy reported in a world class middle-distance athlete after 9 months of added training (5%, 17) but also with the improved running economy in a large group of subjects with different training backgrounds after a 6 months training program of long-distance running (10%; 54). Furthermore, Franch et al. (26) have reported significant improvements in running economy (3.0-3.1%) after 6 weeks of either exhaustive distance training or long-interval training 3 times/week in recreational runners, but not after short-interval training.

It may take more years of serious training to develop a good running economy than to attain each individual's maximal level of $\dot{V}O_2$-max. In a study by Svedenhag & Sjödin (67), ten young and well-trained elite runners (belonging to the Swedish National Team) with judged capacity for performance improvements were followed with regular treadmill tests during one year (January to next January). Of these, 5 were middle-distance runners (mean age 21.2 yrs) and 5 long-distance runners (22.6 yrs). From the competitive season preceding to the one following this test year, the 1500 m time improved from 3:45.0 to 3:40.8 min:s, but 800 m time was essentially unchanged (1:50) (middle-distance runners), and 5000 m time improved from 14:11 to 13:43 min:s (long-distance runners). The $\dot{V}O_2$-max significantly rose from winter to the competitive summer season (74.2 to 77.4 ml•kg^{-1}•min^{-1}; +4.5%). To some part (+1.3%) this was due to a slightly lower body mass during the competitive season. Following winter, the $\dot{V}O_2$-max was almost back to the starting level. In this study running economy at 15 and 20 km/h were determined. A different training response than for $\dot{V}O_2$-max was obtained. The running economy (ml•kg^{-1}•min^{-1}) successively improved during the test year and was between 3-4% lower at the last compared to the first test occasion (specified running velocities). For $\dot{V}O_2$ at 20 km/h ($\dot{V}O_2$-20), this improvement in running economy was significant. There was no change in body mass from a year-to-year basis. Furthermore, in a larger group of elite runners who were followed for 22 months, successive and significant improvements in both $\dot{V}O_2$-15 and $\dot{V}O_2$-20 were found (67). All runners had been familiarised with and tested on the treadmill at least once before commencing the study. Thus, these data suggest a slow but successive improvement in running economy in these elite runners. At the same time, the $\dot{V}O_2$-max was unchanged from year to year (comparisons for the same month). This suggests that it may take longer time to improve the running economy than it takes to reach each individual's maximal obtainable level of $\dot{V}O_2$-max (which in itself may take several years of hard rational training). This could at least partly explain improving performance levels in runners who already have been training for many years.

Thus, even though conclusive scientific data in this area is lacking, it would seem that the differences in running economy between individuals as discussed above is both being due to long-term training effects and to inherent capacities in the first place.

Regarding tapering, Houmard et al. (33) found that a 7-day high-intensity taper improved 5-km performance by 3% and running economy by 6% in a group of 8 highly trained distance runners. The tapering involved an 85% reduction in weekly training volume and daily high-intensity interval workouts at about 100% $\dot{V}O_2$-max. This is in contrast to 1-4 weeks of low-intensity tapering which in earlier studies was unable to improve the running economy (32, 39).

Up/downhill running

The statements above regarding the proper mode of relating $\dot{V}O_2$ to body mass during running preferentially relate to the near *level* running situation. With steep uphill running, during which the body mass is more actively transported against the gravitation, the oxygen uptake may at least theoretically be more closely related to kg^1 than to $kg^{0.75}$. In contrast, during downhill running the $\dot{V}O_2$-submax is lower than for level running and may usually not be a limiting factor (36, 59). Instead, biomechanical factors may be more important as both the maximal speed and maximal stride length may be higher with downhill running at modest negative grades (36). Coming back to power functions, it may thus be seen that the relationship of $\dot{V}O_2$ to body mass may be altered in a rather complicated manner during different parts of a hilly terrain or road racing course. Consequently, this could partly explain the smaller but nonetheless clear performance fluctuations which are known to occur between athletes within such races.

Temperature

The effects of environmental temperature on exercise $\dot{V}O_2$-submax (not properly studied on just running economy) is a complex matter and with different results in the literature. Principally, there may be two opposing effects with an increased core temperature causing 1) increased energy requirements for peripheral circulation, increased sweat gland activity and hyperventilation as well as 2) possible increases in mechanical and/or metabolic efficiency in the musculature (for ref, see 7, 42). It is therefore possible that $\dot{V}O_2$-submax is reduced slightly as muscle temperature is moderately increased but eventually increases as the mechanisms involved in heat dissipation are activated to a greater extent, as discussed by Bailey & Pate (7). It is also conceivable that the running economy may improve with heat acclimatisation due to the corresponding increase in plasma volume.

Air & wind

Obviously, running economy is dependent on air resistance and on wind. On a calm day, the added $\dot{V}O_2$-max due to the air resistance should increase with the cube of the running velocity (58). The actual figures differ somewhat but it has been calculated that the air resistance amounts to 8% of the total energy cost of running when performing a 5000 m run (58) or to 4 and 2% of the $\dot{V}O_2$-max in middle-distance and marathon running, respectively (23). That may explain why only the superior runner may choose an offensive tactic of being a front runner for a whole race and still can be expected to succeed in winning.

Fatigue

As indicated earlier in the variability section, 30 min maximal runs (level running) in at least moderately trained runners have not been shown to produce any significant changes in running economy when tested 1, 2 and 4 days after the run (44, 49). Thus, fatigue in the days following a single exhaustive run may not include changes in the running economy. On the other hand, there are now several studies that have indicated an impaired running economy *within* a single long exercise bout (28, 29, 79). Xu & Montgomery (79) studied the running economy at 3.13 and 3.80 $m \cdot s^{-1}$ in 14 long-distance runners before and after 90-min runs at either 65 or 80% of $\dot{V}O_2$-max. They found increases in $\dot{V}O_2$-submax expressed both as $l \cdot min^{-1}$ and $ml \cdot kg^{-1} \cdot min^{1}$ after the 90-min runs (recalculated as $ml \cdot kg^{-0.75} \cdot min^{-1}$ the increase was 3.7-4.3% after the 65% $\dot{V}O_2$-max run and 5.7-7.8% after the 80% $\dot{V}O_2$-max run). Guezennec et al. (28) compared the running economy at race pace in 11 athletes during a 10-km run in a triathlon (i.e. after 1.5-km swimming and 40-km cycling) with the running economy during a single 10-km control run at the same pace. The running economy was significantly impaired in the 10-km triathlon run with a 7% higher $\dot{V}O_2$-submax (in $ml \cdot kg^{-1} \cdot min^{-1}$). Due to a greater loss in body mass during the triathlon, the corresponding difference in $ml \cdot kg^{-0.75} \cdot min^{-1}$ was 6%. Lastly, Hausswirth et al. (29) studied 7 athletes performing 3 experimental trials; a 2h 15 min triathlon, a 2 h 15 min marathon where the athletes ran the last 45 min at the same speed as during the triathlon run, and a 45 min isolated run at the same speed. They found higher energy cost of running during marathon than during the triathlon run (3.2%) (equal body mass losses in these two exercise modes). The energy cost of running during the latter part of the marathon and during the triathlon was also clearly higher than during the isolated run (about 12% higher cost during the marathon).

The reason for this fatigue effect on the running economy is likely multifactorial. For example, altered biomechanical factors (such as a decreased stride length), increased motor unit recruitment due to glycogen depletion and/or muscle damage, and increased ventilation could all have contributed to the increase in $\dot{V}O_2$-submax in the studies cited above. Also metabolic events have been suggested to play a role, such as an increased fat oxidation with a resultant supposed increase in $\dot{V}O_2$. However, in one study by Morgan et al. (44), the respiratory exchange ratio was slightly but significantly lowered 1 and 2 days after an exhaustive run without any change in running economy. The role of increased fat oxidation for $\dot{V}O_2$-submax thus does not seem to be a major factor in this regard.

Ventilation

Ventilation may be speculated to influence running economy. Thus, the work of ventilation has been found to constitute to up to 6-7% of the total oxygen cost of exercise (41). Furthermore, voluntary hyperpnoea at rest, which increases V_E from 70 to 100 l•min^{-1}, has been found to enhance $\dot{V}O_2$ by 122 ml•min^{-1} (15). If training is able to decrease the work of breathing at a specific running velocity, for instance due to a decreased muscle lactic acid production, this could at least theoretically contribute to an improved running economy (7). Franch et al. (26) also reported a correlation between improvements in running economy and reductions in pulmonary ventilation after an intense run training program in recreational runners. However, more studies are needed before any good estimations on the importance of ventilation can be made.

Step length

With increasing running velocity, there is both an increased step length and an increased step frequency. In elite runners, at least in the 15-18 km•h^{-1} velocity range, the increase in step length may be much more pronounced (15-16%) than the corresponding increase in step frequency (3-4%; 69). For a given running velocity, there is for every individual a U-shaped relationship between step length and running economy and thus an optimal combination range of step length/step frequency at which the $\dot{V}O_2$-submax is at its lowest (34). This optimal combination range, which does not seem to be readily altered with short-term training (6), is mostly self-selected by the runner (13, 34). However, uneconomical freely chosen step lengths in recreational runners have also been shown (47). This self-selection of step lengths may at least partly be related to elastic components (see below) since Taylor (70) has indicated that the speeds and step frequencies selected by animals (and presumably humans) during locomotion are those where storage and recovery of elastic energy are maximised.

In contrast, across different individuals, there is no relationship between step length and running economy (at 3.6 m•s^{-1}; 74), not even when expressed as ml•kg$^{-0.75}$•min^{-1} (69). Anthropometric variables may not at all (recreational runners; 14) or to a very small extent contribute to the chosen step length (positive relationship of step length to body mass and stature, and negative relationship to the leg length/stature quotient in elite runners; 69).

Inflexibility/elastic components

Training of flexibility is often advocated in athletes as a means to reduce the risk of injury and to improve performance and/or recovery. Regarding the effect on performance, this may be a truth with modification as has been indicated in some studies. Thus, Gleim et al. (27) studied 11 measures of trunk and lower limb flexibility in a mixed group of 100 subjects and related the combined score of these measures to the economy of walking and running ($\dot{V}O_2$-submax; in ml•kg^{-1}•min^{-1}). They found that the "tightest" third had significantly lower $\dot{V}O_2$-submax than the "loosest" third, over velocities from 1.79 to 3.13 m•s^{-1}. Craib et al. (19) studied the association between nine measures of limb and trunk flexibility and running economy at 4.13 m•s^{-1} (in ml•kg^{-1}•min^{-1}) in 19 well-trained male sub-elite distance runners who were properly accommodated to treadmill running. The results suggested that inflexibility in hip (standing external hip rotation) and calf regions (dorsiflexion) of the musculoskeletal system was associated with an improved running economy (R^2 when both factors were included was 0.47). This may be in line with the findings of Williams & Cavanagh (74) who noted that runners with the poorest running economy had a significantly less mechanical energy transfer between the legs and the trunk when running at 3.6 m•s^{-1} than runners with better running economy. Also, Heise et al. (30) found a trend towards greater leg muscle coactivation during the stance phase in more economical runners. This was thought to be directly related to joint stiffness, which in turn may be translated to a greater elastic energy return from muscle and tendons contributing to the propulsive stage of the stance phase.

It may thus be hypothesised that besides the observable mechanical work (see below), the elastic components in the running musculature may be of importance (10). As a further example, a 12-week period of additional hill training with "bounce" running was found to improve the running economy in a group of 11 well-trained marathon runners, an effect that was suggested to be related to the development of elastic components with increased storage and return of elastic energy (68). Another interesting study in this context is that of Westblad et al. (72). They had nine male elite 800-5000 m runners completing a test of 100 repetitive maximal eccentric and 100 concentric knee extensor actions (at $90°•s^{-1}$) were peak torque and work were measured.

This was compared with the running economy (in $ml•kg^{-0.75}•min^{-1}$ as well as $ml•kg^{-1}•min^{-1}$) at three different submaximal running velocities. Eccentric total work was found to be inversely related to $\dot{V}O_2$-submax at all three running velocities investigated, with R^2 values for $ml•kg^{-0.75}•min^{-1}$ ranging between 0.48 to 0.59. Thus, the greater eccentric total work in the quadriceps femoris muscle, the better the running economy. Although it is a small study, this effect of the eccentric total work capacity may be speculated to be due to a better ability to store elastic energy.

Thus, from several different studies with different approaches it seems that the elastic components in the running musculature and tendons may be of great importance for the running economy.

Other biomechanical factors

The running economy may be related to the sum of several individual factors related primarily to body structure or running mechanics. Thus, in an extensive investigation by Williams & Cavanagh (74) of 31 recreational runners (running speed 3.6 $m•s^{-1}$), the most economical group of runners were found to have lower force peak at heel strike, greater shank angle with vertical at foot strike (i.e. a more rearfoot striking pattern), smaller maximal plantar flexion angle following the toe off, greater forward trunk lean, and lower minimum velocity of a point on the knee during foot contact. A multiple linear regression model could account for 54% of the variation in aerobic demand. In another study in 14 elite female runners (75; running speed 3.83 and 4.13 $m•s^{-1}$) significant correlations were found between running economy and angle at maximal knee extension near toe-off, maximal knee flexion velocity, maximal dorsiflexion angle and maximal dorsiflexion velocity. Heise et al. (30) studied nine well-trained runners with EMG characteristics of bi-articular leg muscles at a running velocity of 4.13 m•s⁻¹. They found runners with better running economy to have a significantly earlier onset of m. rectus femoris activation and a shorter coactivation of hamstring - m. gastrocnemius during the swing phase.

In reviewing the field, Anderson (1) concluded that several biomechanical factors and anthropometric dimensions may be related to a better running economy, including those listed in Table 3. However, relationships have generally been found to be weak and to some extent inconsistent (e.g. 37). Furthermore, the relative importance of specific factors is very difficult to study/quantitate; the sum of many factors may on the other hand be difficult to interpret. It may well be that each runner has adapted rather optimally to his/her specific/unique com-

Table 3. Some factors related to better running economy in runners. From 1.

Biomechanical factors
- Low vertical oscillation of body centre of mass
- More acute knee angle during swing
- Less range of motion but greater angular velocity of plantar flexion during toe-off
- Arm motion of smaller amplitude
- Low peak ground reaction forces
- Faster rotation of shoulders in the transverse plane
- Greater angular excursion of the hips and shoulders about the polar axis in the transverse plane.

Anthropometric dimensions
- Average or slightly smaller height for men but slightly greater than average height for women
- High ponderal index and ectomorphic or ectomesomorphic physique
- Low percentage body fat
- Leg morphology which distributes mass closer to the hip joint
- Narrow pelvis
- Smaller than average feet.

bination of biomechanical set-up. Making inter-individual comparisons, especially when many biomechanical factors are added together, could therefore potentially be misleading. Earlier studies have also expressed running economy as $ml \cdot kg^{-1} \cdot min^{-1}$ which, according to the discussion above, may not be the proper way to do. Further studies are therefore needed.

Gender

In a substantial part of studies comparing running economy ($ml \cdot kg^{-1} \cdot min^{-1}$) between the sexes, better values in men than in women have been reported (46). Biomechanical gender differences have been put forward as a possible cause of such a difference in running economy. However, the difference in running economy may to a great extent, or perhaps even fully, be explained by body mass differences between the sexes. Thus, the greater body masses of male runners will in a relatively way decrease $\dot{V}O_2$-submax expressed as $ml \cdot kg^{-1} \cdot min^{-1}$, but not as $ml \cdot kg^{-0.75} \cdot min^{-1}$. In fact, when looking at performance-matched male and female marathon runners, the women were actually found to have a better running economy (in $ml \cdot kg^{-0.75} \cdot min^{-1}$) than the men (31). In terms of performance, this partly compensated for the lower $\dot{V}O_2$-max (also in $ml \cdot kg^{-0.75} \cdot min^{-1}$) in this group of female runners.

Another gender aspect is what happens to the running economy during the menstrual cycle phase. Williams & Krahenbuhl (78) studied eight eumenorrheic moderately-trained female runners while running at treadmill speeds initially corresponding to 55 and 80% of $\dot{V}O_2$-max. They found running economy at 80% $\dot{V}O_2$-max to be significantly poorer (higher $\dot{V}O_2$-submax) during the mid-luteal than during the early follicular phase, while no significant difference was seen at 55% $\dot{V}O_2$-max. This effect was thought to be independent of changes in ventilatory drive or mood state.

Age

For more than 40 years it has been known that with increasing age and body mass during growth, both $\dot{V}O_2$-submax and $\dot{V}O_2$-max (in $ml \cdot kg^{-1} \cdot min^{-1}$) will decrease (2). The reasons for this were earlier not well understood. Regarding the $\dot{V}O_2$-submax, several factors have been suggested to explain the lower running economy in children, including higher stride frequency, immature running biomechanics, lesser utilisation of muscle elastic energy, a different substrate utilisation and less efficient ventilation. However, calculations made in the above mentioned longitudinal study of Sjödin & Svedenhag (62) favoured oxygen uptake being related to $kg^{-0.75}$ instead of kg^{-1} and in this case the $\dot{V}O_2$-submax will remain unchanged in both the untrained and trained boys during growth. For the untrained boys also the $\dot{V}O_2$-max will be unchanged but in trained boys it will increase (as would be expected in adults). Further support for the use of body mass power functions of 0.67 – 0.80 has come from studies of peak $\dot{V}O_2$ in different groups of prepubertal, circumpubertal and adult males and females (71).

Psychological/ mood state

The psychological state may be related to the running economy, at least in an indirect way. Williams et al. (77) studied ten runners five times a week for 4 weeks and correlated the running economy to the total score and different measures of the Profile of Mood States (POMS). They found no relations in the whole group of runners but a significant *within-subject* correlation of $r=0.88$, mainly related to the tension score. Thus, in the weeks with lower scores, there was a better running economy. In reviewing the few studies done at that time, Crews (20) concluded that relaxation techniques, especially stress management techniques, appear to improve running economy but that biofeedback procedures that may change heart rate or ventilatory responses do not change running economy. Since then some more studies have been added. When investigating 18 competitive male distance runners at 4.13 $m{\cdot}s^{-1}$, Martin et al. (38) found the most economical runners to be the ones that habitually directed attention inwards. It was hypothesised that this could reduce anxiety which, in turn, could contribute to a better running economy. Lastly, Smith et al. (64) studied 36 distance runners and found that the most economical runners reported less dissociation use and more use of relaxation than did the least economical runners. While all these findings are intriguing, longitudinal studies aiming at changing psychological strategies during running and their effect on running economy are still missing.

Miscellaneous

Other factors such as muscle strength in the running musculature and torso (for more effective muscle stabilisation during running) and factors related to muscle energy production and oxidative capacity may, at least in theory, also contribute to the described variation in running economy.

Concluding remarks

Running economy is obviously one important factor determining running capacity in endurance events, but it should be expressed in a proper way, i.e. in $ml \cdot kg^{-0.75} \cdot min^{-1}$. Given test conditions are well controlled, running economy seems to be a quite robust measure. It may, however, change within a single exercise bout or with long-term training. Of the many factors that may determine running economy, the ability to store/use elastic energy in the running musculature and tendons may be especially important.

References

1. Anderson T. Biomechanics and running economy. *Sports Med.* 22:76-89, 1996.
2. Åstrand P-O. *Experimental studies of physical working capacity in relation to sex and age.* Thesis, Munksgaard, Copenhagen. 1952.
3. Åstrand P-O. New records in human power. *Nature* 176: 922-923, 1955.
4. Åstrand P-O, Rodahl K. *Textbook of Work Physiology.* Chapter 9: Body dimensions and muscular exercise. New York, McGraw-Hill, 1986.
5. Alexander RM, Jayes AS, Maloiy GMO, Wathuta EM. Allometry of the leg muscles of mammals. *J Zool Lond* 194: 539-552, 1981.
6. Bailey SP, Messier SP. Variations in stride length and running economy in male novice runners subsequent to a seven-week training program. *Int J Sports Med* 12: 299-304, 1991.
7. Bailey SP, Pate RR. Feasibility of improving running economy. *Sports Med* 12:228-236, 1991.
8. Bangsbo J, Gollnick P D, Graham T E, Juel C, Kiens B, Mizuno M, Saltin B. Anaerobic energy production and O_2 deficit-debt relationship during exhaustive exercise in humans. *J Physiol* 422: 539-559, 1990.
9. Bergh U, Sjödin B, Forsberg A, Svedenhag J. The relationship between body mass and oxygen uptake during running in humans. *Med Sci Sports Exerc* 23: 205-211, 1991.

10. Bosco G, Montanari R, Ribacchi P et al. Relationship between the efficiency of muscular work during jumping and the energetics or running. *Eur J Appl Physiol* 56: 138-143, 1987.

11. Bourdin M, Pastene J, Germain M, Lacour JR. Influence of training, sex, age and body mass on the energy cost of running. *Eur J Appl Physiol* 66: 439-444, 1993.

12. Brisswalter J, Legros P. Daily stability in energy cost of running, respiratory parameters and stride rate among well-trained middle distance runners. *Int J Sports Med* 15:238-241, 1994.

13. Cavanagh PR, Williams KR. The effect of stride length variation on oxygen uptake during distance running. *Med Sci Sports Exerc* 14:30-35, 1982.

14. Cavanagh PR, Kram R. Stride length in distance running: velocity, body dimensions, and added mass effects. *Med Sci Sports Exerc* 21:467-479, 1989.

15. Coast JR, Krause KM. Relationship of oxygen consumption and cardiac output to work of breathing. *Med Sci Sports Exerc* 25:335-340, 1993.

16. Conley DL, Krahenbuhl GS. Running economy and distance running performance of highly trained athletes. *Med Sci Sports Exerc* 12: 357-360, 1980.

17. Conley DL, Krahenbuhl GS, Burkett LN, Millar AL. Following Steve Scott: Physiological changes accompanying training. *Physician and Sports Med* 12:103-106, 1984.

18. Costill DL, Thomason H, Roberts E. Fractional utilization of the aerobic capacity during distance running. *Med Sci Sports* 5: 248-252, 1973.

19. Craib MW, Mitchell VA, Fields KB, Cooper TR, Hopewell R, Morgan DW. The association between flexibility and running economy in sub-elite male distance runners. *Med Sci Sports Exerc* 28:737-743, 1996.

20. Crews DJ. Psychological state and running economy. *Med Sci Sports Exerc* 24:475-482, 1992.

21. Daniels JT, Yarbrough RA, Foster C. Changes in VO_2-max and running performance with training. *Eur J Appl Physiol* 39:249-254, 1978.

22. Daniels J, Daniels N. Running economy of elite male and elite female runners. *Med Sci Sports Exerc* 24:483-489, 1992.

23. Davies CTM. Effects of wind assistance and resistance on the forward motion of a runner. *J Appl Physiol* 48:702-709, 1980.

24. Davies CTM, Thompson MW. Aerobic performance of female marathon and male ultramarathon athletes. *Eur J Appl Physiol* 41:233-245, 1979.

25. von Döbeln W. Maximal oxygen intake, body size, and total hemoglobin in normal man. *Acta Physiol Scand* 38: 193-199, 1956.

26. Franch J, Madsen K, Djurhuus MS, Pedersen PK. Improved running economy following intensified training correlates with reduced ventilatory demands. *Med Sci Sports Exerc* 30:1250-1256, 1998.

27. Gleim GW, Stachenfeld NS, Nicholas JA. The influence of flexibility on the economy of walking and jogging. *J Orthopaedic Res* 8:814-823, 1990.

28. Guezennec CY, Vallier JM, Bigard AX, Durey A. Increase in energy cost of running at the end of a triathlon. *Eur J Appl Physiol* 73:440-445, 1996.

29. Hausswirth C, Bigard AX, Guezennec CY. Relationships between running mechanics and energy cost of running at the end of a triathlon and a marathon. *Int J Sports Med* 18:330-339, 1997.

30. Heise GD, Morgan DW, Hough H, Craib M. Relationships between running economy and temporal EMG characteristics of bi-articular leg muscles. *Int J Sports Med* 17:128-133, 1996.

31. Helgerud J. Maximal oxygen uptake, anaerobic threshold and running economy in women and men with similar performances level in marathons. *Eur J Appl Physiol* 68: 155-161, 1994.

32. Houmard JA, Kirwan JP, Flynn MG, Mitchell JB. Effects of reduced training on submaximal and maximal running responses. In *J Sports Med* 10:30-33, 1989.

33. Houmard JA, Scott BK, Justice CL, Chenier TC. The effects of taper on performance in distance runners. *Med Sci Sports Exerc* 26:624-631, 1994.

34. Högberg P. How do stride length and stride frequency influence the energy-output during running? *Arbeitsphysiologie* 14:437-441, 1952.

35. Lake MJ, Cavanagh PR. Six weeks of training does not change running mechanics or improve running economy. *Med Sci Sports Exerc* 28:860-869, 1996.

36. Liefeldt G, Noakes TD, Dennis SC. Oxygen delivery does not limit peak running speed during incremental downhill running to exhaustion. *Eur J Appl Physiol* 64:493-496, 1992.

37. Martin PE, Heise GD, Morgan DW. Interrelationships between mechanical power, energy transfers, and walking and running economy. *Med Sci Sports Exerc* 25:508-515, 1993.

38. Martin JJ, Craib M, Mitchell V. The relationships of anxiety and self-attention to running economy in competitive male distance runners. *J Sports Sci* 13:371-376, 1995.

39. McConell GK, Costill DL, Widrick JJ, Hickey MS, Tanaka H, Gastin PB. Reduced training volume and intensity maintain aerobic capacity but not performance in distance runners. *Int J Sports Med* 14:33-37, 1993.

40. McMahon T. Size and shape in biology. Elastic criteria impose limits on biological proportions, and consequently on metabolic rates. *Science* 174: 1201-1204, 1973.

41. Milic-Emili G, Petit JM, Deroanne R. Mechanical work of breathing during exercise in trained and untrained subjects. *J Appl Physiol* 17:43-46, 1962.

42. Morgan DW, Martin PE, Krahenbuhl GS. Factors affecting running economy. *Sports Med* 7:310-330, 1989a.

43. Morgan DW, Baldini FD, Martin PE, Kohrt WM. Ten kilometer performance and predicted velocity at VO_2-max among well-trained male runners. *Med Sci Sports Exerc* 21: 78-83, 1989b.

44. Morgan DW, Martin PE, Baldini FD, Krahenbuhl GS. Effects of a prolonged maximal run on running economy and running mechanics. *Med Sci Sports Exerc* 22:834-840, 1990.

45. Morgan DW, Martin PE, Krahenbuhl GS, Baldini FD. Variability in running economy and mechanics among trained male runners. *Med Sci Sports Exerc* 23:378-383, 1991.

46. Morgan DW, Craib M. Physiological aspects of running economy. *Med Sci Sports Exerc* 24: 456-461, 1992.

47. Morgan D, Martin P, Craib M, Caruso C, Clifton R, Hopewell R. Effect of step length optimization on the aerobic demand of running. *J Appl Physiol* 77: 245-251, 1994.

48. Morgan DW, Bransford DR, Costill DL, Daniels JT, Howley ET, Krahenbuhl GS. Variation in the aerobic demand of running among trained and untrained subjects. *Med Sci Sports Exerc* 27:404-409, 1995.

49. Morgan DW, Strohmeyer HS, Daniels JT, Beaudoin CC, Craib MW, Borden RA, Greer PJ, Burleson CL. Short-term changes in 10-km race pace aerobic demand and gait mechanics following a bout of high-intensity distance running. *Eur J Appl Physiol* 73:267-272, 1996.

50. Myers M, Steudel K. Effect of limb mass and its distribution on the energetic cost of running. *J Exp Biol* 116:363-373, 1985.

51. Nevill AM. The need to scale for differences in body size and mass: an explanation of Kleiber's 0.75 mass exponent. *J Appl Physiol* 77: 2870-2873, 1994.

52. Noakes TD. Implications of exercise testing for prediction of athletic performance: a contemporary perspective. *Med Sci Sports Exerc* 20: 319-330,1988.

53. Padilla S, Bourdin M, Barthélémy JC, Lacour JR. Physiological correlates of middle-distance running performance. A comparative study between men and women. *Eur J Appl Physiol* 65: 561-566, 1992.

54. Patton JF, Vogel JA. Cross-sectional and longitudinal evaluations of an endurance training program. *Med Sci Sports* 9:100-103, 1977.

55. di Prampero PE, Atchou G, Brückner J-C, Moia C. The energetics of endurance running. *Eur J Appl Physiol* 55: 259-266, 1986.

56. Pate RR, Macera CA, Bailey SP, Bartoli WP, Power KE. Physiological, anthropometric and training correlates of running economy. *Med Sci Sports Exerc* 24: 1128-1133, 1992.

57. Pereira MA, Freedson PS. Intraindividual variation of running economy in highly trained and moderately trained males. *Int J Sports Med* 18:118-124, 1997.

58. Pugh LGCE. Oxygen intake in track and treadmill running with observations on the effect of air resistance. *J Physiol* 207:823-835, 1970.

59. Robergs RA, Wagner DR, Skemp KM. Oxygen consumption and energy expenditure of level versus downhill running. *J Sports Med Phys Fitness* 37:168-174, 1997.

60. Robinson S, Edwards HT, Dill DB. New records in human power. *Science* 83: 409-410, 1937.

61. Sjödin B, Svedenhag J. Applied physiology of marathon running. *Sports Med* 2: 83-99, 1985.

62. Sjödin B, Svedenhag J. Oxygen uptake during running as related to body mass in circumpubertal boys: a longitudinal study. *Eur J Appl Physiol* 65: 150-157, 1992.

63. Sjödin B, Jacobs I, Svedenhag J. Changes in onset of blood lactate accumulation (OBLA) and muscle enzymes after training at OBLA. *Eur J Appl Physiol* 49:45-57, 1982.

64. Smith AL, Gill DL, Crews DJ, Hopewell R, Morgan DW. Attentional strategy use by experienced distance runners: physiological and psychological effects. *Res Quart Exer Sport* 66:142-150, 1995.

65. Svedenhag J. Maximal and submaximal oxygen uptake during running: how should body mass be accounted for? *Scand J Med Sci Sports* 5:175-180, 1995.

66. Svedenhag J, Sjödin B. Maximal and submaximal oxygen uptakes and blood lactate levels in elite male middle- and long-distance runners. *Int J Sports Med* 5: 255-261, 1984.

67. Svedenhag J, Sjödin B. Physiological characteristics of elite male runners in and off season. *Can J Appl Spt Sci* 10: 127-133, 1985.

68. Svedenhag J. Endurance conditioning. In: *Endurance in Sport. Vol II of the Encyclopaedia of Sports Medicine, an IOC. Medical Commission Publication,* (eds. J. Shephard & P-O Åstrand). Blackwell Scientific Publications, Oxford 1992: pp 290-297.

69. Svedenhag J, Sjödin B. Body-mass-modified running economy and step length in elite male middle- and long-distance runners. *Int J Sports Med* 15: 305-310, 1994.

70. Taylor R. Force development during sustained locomotion: a determinant of gait, speed and metabolic power. *J Exp Biol* 115:253-262, 1985.

71. Welsman JR, Armstrong N, Nevill AM, Winter EM, Kirby BJ. Scaling peak VO_2 for differences in body size. *Med Sci Sports Exerc* 28:259-265, 1996.

72. Westblad P, Svedenhag J, Rolf C. The validity of isokinetic knee extensor endurance measurements with reference to treadmill running capacities. *Int J Sports Med* 17:134-139, 1996.

73. Wilcox AR, Bulbulian R. Changes in running economy relative to VO_2-max during a cross-country season. *J Sports Med* 24:321-326, 1984.

74. Williams KR, Cavanagh PR. Relationship between distande running mechanics, running economy, and performance. *J Appl Physiol* 63: 1236-1245, 1987.

75. Williams KR, Cavanagh PR, Ziff JL. Biomechanical studies of elite female distance runners. *Int J Sports Med* 8: S107-S118, 1987.

76. Williams TJ, Krahenbuhl GS, Morgan DW. Daily variation in running economy of moderately trained male runners. *Med Sci Sports Exerc* 23:944-948, 1991a.

77. Williams TJ, Krahenbuhl GS, Morgan DW. Mood state and running economy in moderately trained male runners. *Med Sci Sports Exerc* 23:727-731, 1991b.

78. Williams TJ, Krahenbuhl GS. Menstrual cycle phase and running economy. *Med Sci Sports Exerc* 29:1609-1618, 1997.

79. Xu F, Montgomery DL. Effect of prolonged exercise at 65 and 80% of VO_2-max on running economy. *Int J Sports Med* 16:309-315, 1995.

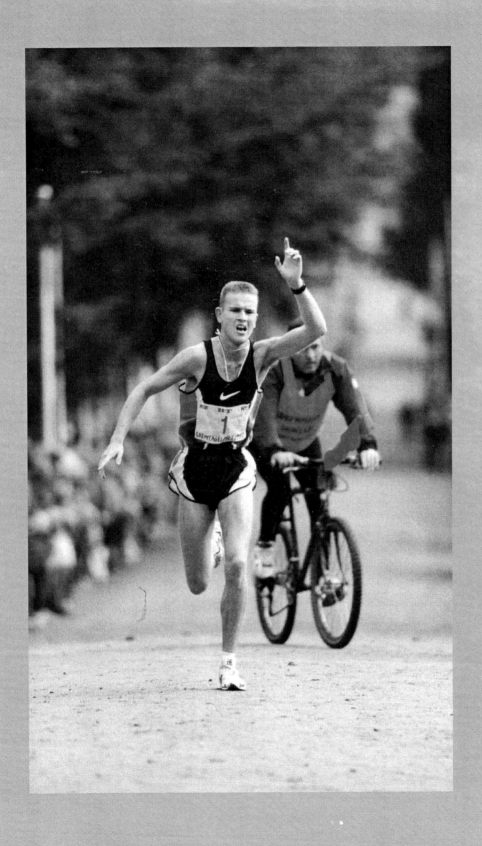

Prevention of overuse injuries in running

Albert Gollhofer

Synopsis

Large epidemiological surveys have indicated that in running the vast majority of overuse injuries is related to the lower limb. In literature most of the problems occurring with overuse injuries in running are attributed to either intrinsic or extrinsic factors. In a „top-down-approach" a brief overview about the most potential risk factors and their possible prophylactic counteracts is given. In order to motivate the physiological implication of the entire system in a „bottom-up-approach" the interaction of man-shoe-surface is described.

Introduction

During the 1970's and 80's running and jogging has developed to become one of the most popular sports disciplines in the world. In line with this trend the number of injuries has increased. Despite the fact that running is considered to be beneficial in lowering the main risk factors of cardio-vascular disease (7), obesity and hypertension (3) the number of orthopaedic problems associated with running gives rise to the question whether or not this type of physical activity is still recommendable or even harmful.

An understanding of the mechanisms through which the most frequent injuries are caused is essential in the evaluation of preventive provisions. Studying the aetiology of running injuries leads to adequate knowledge to reduce the major and most common risk factors. However, with respect to the literature already the attempt to define the basic terms – "overuse", "prevention", and even "running" and "injury" –produces more questions than answers.

Prevention cannot be related to one single, monocausal aspect. Prevention must consider the entire complex of the kinetic chain. The history of individual predisposition has to be recognised and prevention needs to be based on a physical examination of the athletes or participants (8). There is an ongoing extensive debate about the validation criteria of such examinations. Static versus dynamic testing, treadmill versus free running, inter– versus intraindividual comparison, all these methodological aspects are debated in the literature with respect to their apparent advantage.

Overuse is not a unique occurrence. Overuse appears largely different in highly trained athletes and in occasionally jogging overweights. Overuse injuries may be characterised as a chronic dysfunction as the result of a cumulative microtraumatic loading of the tissue; or they may happen as an acute type, especially in high intensity running.

A further aspect in the existing discrepancy can be seen in the various definitions of "injury". Regarding the epidemiological reports in the literature running injuries are summarised as those "serious enough for training reduction" or for "training stop" or "work time loss" or "even pain for more than 10 days". Moreover there exits a high interrelation between the location, the severity of injury and the runners experience (15).

The final problem is the definition of a "runner". In the literature running injuries are assigned to each type of problem occurring during locomotion. A runner may be an orienteer, a marathon runner, a sprinter or even an elite hurdle specialist, he may be experienced or not, young or old.

The purpose of this contribution is to describe potential preventive measures that are effective enough to reduce or avoid overuse injuries in running. On the basis of the published material, two strategies can be distinguished:
a) in a "top-down approach" the incidence of injuries is examined statistically, reflecting the potential risk of the runner, the running and the environmental situation (13).
b) in a "bottom-up model" the physiological implication of an individual runner is reflected in the interaction of the man, the shoe and the surface (5).

Epidemiology – incidence of injuries

Large epidemiological surveys about running injuries have been published in the last decade.

Analysing a total number of 15212 injuries Steinbrück (20) demonstrated that the lower extremity is the most injured body area in sports. More than two third of all injuries are injuries of the knee or ankle joint (Figure 1).

A direct comparison of the incidence of injuries in running and in ball sports from Segesser (19) reveals that in running, the tendineous structures are much more affected than in ball sports. This high rate, observed especially in the lower leg, is a result mainly due to Achilles tendon problems. Based on a statistical survey from 1903 injuries from running and from 1664 injuries from ballsports, the shank and knee problems due to ligamentous and tendineous deficits or obvious. Whereas in ball sport injuries the tendon injuries of the shank area are rather rare this source of incidence is most frequent in running.

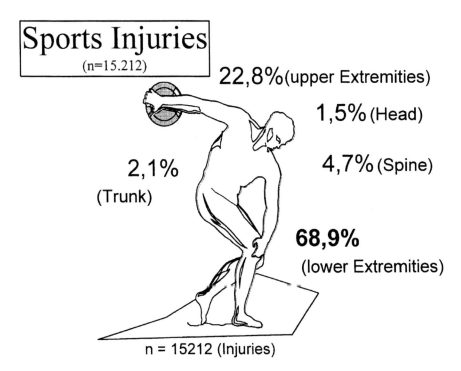

Figure 1. Distributed frequency of sport injuries. Data from 20.

Results from two Dutch studies suggested that the total risk in running is between 3.5 and 5.5 incidences per 1000h of running (4, 16). Thus, on the basis of the Marti et al (15) study running injuries occur about 2-2,5 times less frequent than do injuries in all others sports, and even about 6 times less than ski injuries.

Approaches – Aetiology of injuries

It has been claimed (13) that the majority of overuse injuries are caused by intrinsic (age, gender, body alignment, muscular system, etc.) and extrinsic (footware, training, heat, cold, etc.) factors. The multifactorial causation is analysed statistically based on the assumptions that intrinsic (i.e. primary and secondary) dysfunctions and extrinsic (i.e. environmental) factors are both important.

In a significant contribution van Mechelen (16) reviewed the current literature to analyse whether the runner – the running or the environment have potential influence to explain overuse injuries. By means of multiple analysis of variance, factor regression and other statistical approaches, the assessment of the risk potential of those intrinsic factors has been investigated. In order to discuss the relative importance as potential source of injury a short summary is given in the following chapters for the most important factors.

The runner

Depending on methodological peculiarities and on the statistical model there are reports demonstrating an increasing and a decreasing effect of age on the injury rate. If age is analysed in a multiple step-wise regression, however, it turns out that age is a rather independent factor. Neither age alone nor age associated with experience or with weekly running distance is associated with injury (16).

With respect to running Macintyre et al (14) showed that the most frequent injury in running is related to the knee joint complex, independent of the gender of the subjects.

Gender per se does not represent an important risk factor. It could be hypothesised that body weight has an considerable impact on the incidence rate. If body mass is normalised with body height the body mass index (BMI) should be high in those people, who are subjected more frequently injury. The study, however, produced no statistical effects of BMI and the incidence rate. It must be conceded, however, that the number of runners with an BMI index greater than 30 is probably rather rare!

Malalignments such as different limb length, knee anomalies (knock-knees; bow-legs; patellar deformities) or foot anomalies (varus/valgus etc.) seem in 40% of retrospectively analysed injuries to be one of the injury causes (12). It must be pointed out that the hypothesis that abnormalities are potential risk factors for injury is also reasonable. The question is whether statistical or individual analysis will give the appropriate solution.

Running experience seems to be one of the major factors. It is suggested that long term adaptation of the tissue and of the biomechanics of running leads to a significant reduction of injury rates although bias to the selective problems of the healthier runner must be considered.

The classification of "previous injuries" is not unique in literature. "Old injury" or "repaired tissue failed" is also summarised as well as insufficient rehabilitation. However, it seems that previous injuries are a major factor for running injuries. Therefore prevention must start with management to avoid recurrence of that specific problem.

The running

Running distance or mileage expressed either per week, month or year has only a positive influence on incidence rate if taken absolutely. The relative risk (risk per exposure time), however, is decreased (6, 11). Several authors comment that the frequency of running has a strong influence on injury rate. Although running distance and frequency is strongly interrelated, the study of Marti et al (15) indicated, that in subjects running the same distance either in two, three or four sessions per week, frequency has no significant effect on the probability getting injured.

A classical parameter characterising overuse represents the training error (1) and change of training habits. Powell et al (18) stated that a sudden change in running or training habits increases the incidence rate of injury because of a lack of capacity of the tissue to adapt. Training errors (running too fast, too long or too often) are strong indicators for increased injury probability. Lysholm/Wiklander (12) found that training errors are associated with 60% of all running injuries! For effective prevention the key–question remains to be solved individually: How much is too much?

Environmental systems

There is an ongoing debate about the principal capability of sport or running shoes to influence injury rate. Extensive industrial and scientific projects have been conducted in order to develop the appropriate shoe: shock absorption in the rear part for the heel strikers as well as in the front for the mid or fore foot strikers have been promoted.

On the basis of biomechanical calculations, a single leg is subjected to 60 t per km assuming a strike length of 1,5 m, a contact rate of 670 times per km a body weight 70kg and an average impact loading of 2.5 times body weight. It is evident that a running shoe plays a significant role in shock absorption providing cushioning, support and stability. The construction of a running shoe with these qualities is seen as a major contribution in injury prevention.

Malalignments of the human locomotor system is thought to be correctable by orthodic devices. By means of tape or in-shoe devices it has been demonstrated that the injury rate can be reduced by a factor of two. This effect, however, is most probably biased by the actuality that those runners who a prone to possible injuries tend to apply for orthodics.

In general, cushioning, support and stability are necessary qualities of the shoe material. Injury reduction can be effectively achieved with additional equipment known as orthodic devices. It must, however, be kept in mind, that even the best quality shoe will loose 30-50% of its prevention properties after few hundred kilometres of running (2).

It must be pointed out that this conclusion is the outcome of statistical calculations, expressing the probability of a group or subgroup getting injured. The fact that some of these factors are unclear or even irrelevant for injuries does not mean that they are not unimportant. Epidemiological research is necessary to get an over-all information about that issue. Statistical analysis has some implications for the majority of a group or subgroup of runners.

Man-Shoe-Surface – Interaction

In a "bottom up" strategy some research is focused on the complex entity of the man-the shoe and the surface, in order to investigate the individual responses.

One of the most powerful tools in overuse prevention is a careful and comprehensive screening and testing of the athletes themselves. Whereas in top athletes individual gait analysis and physiological examination should not be a great problem, the situation in lower level runners is controversial. Most of the ligamentous and tendineous problems could be avoided if the runner is inspected carefully before initiation of training. There is, however, not enough data available that gives a clearly indication of what is dangerous or harmful and what is within the physiological limits. There are only few anatomical and biomechanical factors that can be extracted to explain increased injury risks mainly because of the individual variability and because of the flexible adaptability of the locomotor system.

Excessive pronation (hyperpronation) is one of the most frequent problems that is associated with a series of different potentials to cause overuse injuries: Tendinitis at the Achilles tendon, fasciitis on the plantaris as well as lateralisation of the patellar alignment (runners knee) and even shin splints are possible consequences (13).

Therefore, a careful inspection of possible pronation (b-angle) tested either in static or in dynamic situation or is a necessity for everybody prior to training.

In the field of locomotion one assumption is made that there exists an interaction between all components which interfere in generation and control of locomotion (9, 10). Therefore the dependency and interaction of man, shoe and surface is assumed to play an important role which cannot be neglected in a comprehensive study of locomotion.

Man as a biological system utilises all the possibilities for action and reaction to environmental influences. The human neuromuscular system is, however, adaptive with a range of flexibility and variability to achieve appropriate movement pattern. In this respect it should be assumed that not only the intraindividual behaviour is flexible when the conditions are changed, but also the differences in intraindividual comparison should be taken into consideration. A well trained athlete in running, for example, would respond to changes in running conditions in a different manner than a subject with less skill and lower training status.

The neuromuscular system is not only responsible for the regulation of the exertion of forces to produce posture and /or locomotion; additionally it is a control system via several sensory mechanisms which are capable to react through feedback to small disturbances in running cycles or running conditions. Facilitation or reduction of these feedback mechanisms makes it possible for the human locomotor system to meet a great variety of movement conditions by supplying the musculature with adequate contractile and stiffness properties.

The function of the shoes which represent the second component in the chain of interaction, can be explained in two ways. On one hand the shoes transfer the action forces to the ground and on the other hand they mediate the reaction forces from the ground back to the body. Therefore the shoe construction must be oriented on both the physical and physiological requirements of running.

The physical properties of running shoes can also be described in two other ways. First, the shoes should have cushioning properties which suppress high impact forces especially in the early impact phase to protect the skeleton and tendon from extreme loading. Secondly, the characteristics of the shoe should provide support in the various strides under a large number of different running situations. Support combines both the reduction of unphysiological supination and pronation in the stride phases (17), as well as the task to act during the stance phase to overcome the individual load and to help actively in the running cycles. The latter argument, however, can be interpreted in terms of running economy, running performance or even performance potentiation.

The qualities and elasticity characteristics or the running surface may play an important role and may influence to a great deal not only the running technique and running comfort but also the physiological demands to the runner. The variability may range from very hard surfaces, such as asphalt conditions which represent the surface condition in marathon running, to a very soft ground which is mostly found in jogging tracks, consisting of pure soil and sawdust.

Examination of the qualities of running must therefore take into consideration the entire system "man-shoe-surface". All of these three components have their own physical resonance characteristics, but when acting together the "man" must respond physiologically to make the best out of the combination.

All these components which contribute the man-shoe-surface interaction, have their own qualities and quantitative contributions in running. Only a positive interference of all three components will lead to an effective and efficient running pattern.

In the example demonstrated in Figure 2, the comparison of the force and EMG pattern of the same subject running is presented with different shoes. Shoe qualities have a considerable impact on physiological demands: In figure 2, it is shown that with seven different shoes, ranging from very soft to very hard, a considerable alteration in the EMG profile of the lower leg muscle is concommitant. This segmentation of the EMG pattern during the breaking phase is clear and consistent with respect to timing. The individual amplitudes, however, are considerably changed in different conditions.

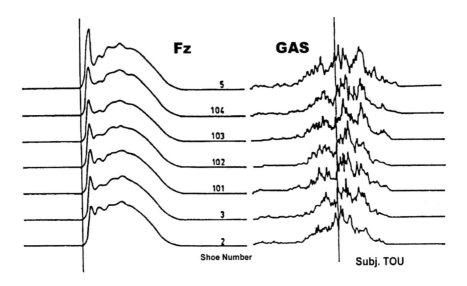

Figure 2. Vertical ground reaction forces and EMG–pattern of m. Gastrocnemius (GAS) of one subject running (5m•s⁻¹) with 7 shoes. From top: the stiffness of the sole construction is decreased. In line with the stiffness characteristics of the shoes the initial peak of the force record emerges. Comparison of the EMG-pattern reveal large alterations in amplitude right after ground contact (vertical line).

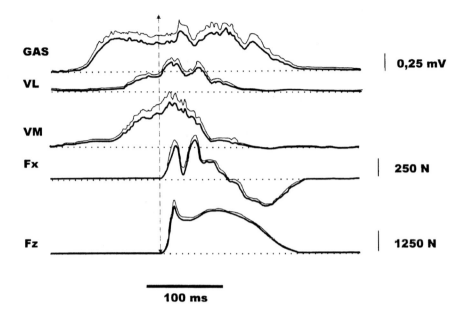

Figure 3. Ground reaction forces and EMG-pattern of leg muscles represented as the grand mean curves (mean (thick line) and standard deviation curve (thin line) of one subject running with constant velocity of 5 m•s^1 with 22 shoes with different stiffness properties. Note that there is a considerable variance in the EMG-patterns whereas in the force records only small variations exist.

In a comprehensive comparison (Figure 3), the differences of 22 shoes were evaluated in one subject running with 5 m•s^1 over a long platform (5). The figures were composed using a statistical method for the grand mean calculation. The individual averages were matched with respect to the onset of ground contact. The dark line represented the mean curve, the thin line the +1 standard deviation of all tested performances. The vertical force component shows variability primarily during the early impact. The variation in the force record can only be expressed in terms of amplitudes and not of time. The activation patterns show little variation in timing of the onset of preactivation, and in the rate of rise of activation. The total amount of electrical input to the muscle however, varied substantially with 30% of the mean value.

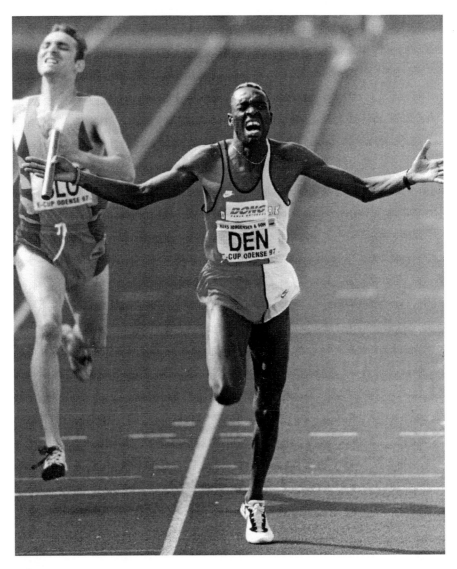

Conclusion

Injury-free running cannot be guaranteed. However, the risk of overuse injury can effectively be minimised. In the general view, a huge amount of research is necessary to elucidate the real potential risk factors. Only controlled studies analysing the distinct roles of these factors will give the necessary help. Before all this effort, a clear and well agreed definition of the basic terms –prevention, overuse, running and injury – is necessary.

In accordance with this, a detailed individual analysis of the entire complex – the man, the shoe and the surface – is an evident prerequisite to assess the biomechanical and physiological adaptability.

Methodologically, a reference frame with clear defined standards is missing to judge positive, non relevant or even harmful influences on an individual basis.

A competent screening of the athlete, adequate training parameters, especially with respect to duration and intensity of the running exercises, are certainly the most powerful preventive measures in reducing overuse injury in running.

In general, it can be recognised that the muscle specific pattern is reproducible in its shape throughout all conditions. This reflects, that the individual pattern is quite stable and that the magnitude is drastically changed in different running conditions with different compliance characteristic.

References

1. Clement, D. B.; Tauton, J. E.; Smart, G. W. & Nicol, K. L. : A survey of overuse running injuries. *Phys. Sports Med.* 9 (5), 47-58, 1981.
2. Cook, S. D.; Brinker, M. R. & Mahlon, P. : Running shoes. Their relation to running injuries. *Sports Med.* 10 (1), 1-8, 1990.
3. Eichner, E. R. : Exercise and heart disease. Epidemiology of the 'exercise hypothesis'. *Am. J. Med.* 75, 1008-23, 1983.
4. Galen van, W.; Diederiks van, J. : *Sportblessures Breed Uitgemeten* (A Population Study on Sport Injuries). De Vrieseborch, Haarlem, The Netherlands, 1990.
5. Gollhofer, A.; Komi, P. V. : Measurement of man-shoe-surface interaction during locomotion. In: *Med. and Sport Science* 26: Karger, Basel, 187-199, 1987.
6. Jacobs, S. J., Berson, B. L. : Injuries to runners: A study of entrants to a 10000 meter race. *Am. J. Sports Med.* 14 (2), 151-5, 1986.
7. Jesse, J. : Hidden Causes of Injury, Prevention and Correction for Running Athletes and Joggers. *The Athletic Press,* Pasadena, CA. 1977
8. Kibler, W. B. : The Sport Preparticipation Fitness Examination. *Human Kinetics,* Illinois, 1990.
9. Komi, P.V.: Physiological and biomechanical correlates of muscle function effects of muscle structure and stretch-shortening cycle on force and speed. *Exercise and Sort Sciences Reviews,* 12, 81-121,1984

10. Komi, P.V.; Hyvärinen,T.; Gollhofer, A.: Man-shoe-surface interaction. Special problems during marathon running. Special problems during marathon running. *Acta Uni. Oul.* 179, 69-72, 1986

11. Koplan, J. P.; Powell, K. E.; Sikes, P. K.; Shirley, R. W. & Campell, C. C. : An epidemiologic study of the benefits and risks of running. *JAMA* 248 (23), 3118-21, 1982.

12. Lysholm, J.; Wiklander, J. : Injuries in runners. *Am. J. Sports Med.* 15 (2), 168-71, 1987.

13. Macintyre, J.; Lloyd-Smith, R. : Overuse Running Injuries. Renström, P. A. F. H. (Ed.): Sports Injuries. Basic Principles of Prevention and Care. *Blackwell Scientific Publications.* 139-160, 1993

14. Macintyre, J. G.; Tauton, J. E.; Clement, D. B.; Lloyd-Smith, D. R.; McKenzie, D. C. & Morrell, R. W. : Running injuries: A clinical surveys of 4173 cases. *Clin. J. Sports Med.* 1 (2), 81-7, 1991.

15. Marti, B.; Vader, J. P.; Minder, E. C. & Abelin, T. : On the epidemiology of running injuries : The 1984 Bern Grand Prix Study. *Am. J. Sports Med.* 16, 285-94, 1988.

16. Mechelen van, W. : *Aetiology and prevention of running injuries.* Thesis, Vrije Universiteit, Amsterdam, 1992.

17. Nigg, B.M.: Biomechanical analysis of ankle and foot movement. *Med. and Science in Sports and Exercise,* 23, 22-29, 1987.

18. Powell, K. E.; Kohl, H. W.; Caspersen, C. J. & Blair, S. N. : An epedimiological perspective on the causes of running injuries. *Phys. Sports Med.* 14 (6), 100-14, 1986.

19. Segesser, B. : Sportschuhe. In: *GOTS-MANUAL Sporttraumatologie.* Verlag Hans Huber, 1997.

20. Steinbrück, K. : Epidemiologie. *GOTS-MANUAL Sporttraumatologie.* Verlag Hans Huber, 1997.

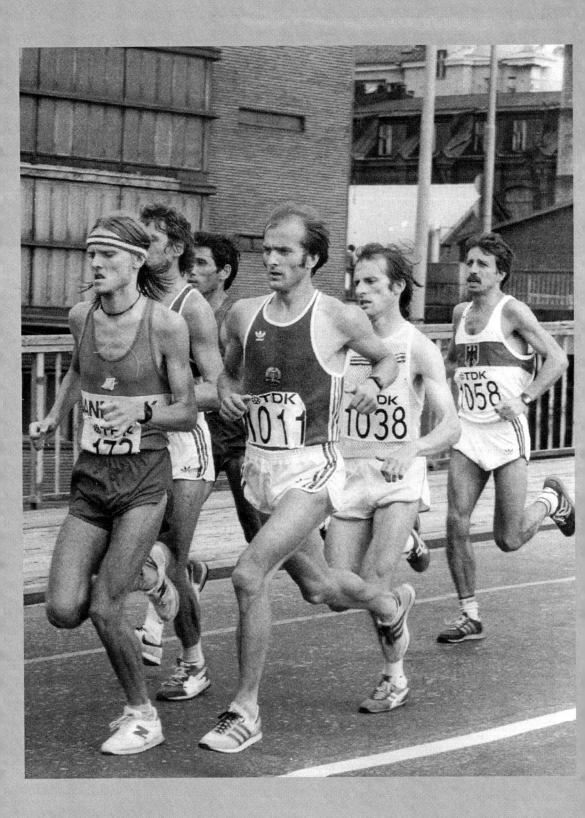

Training principles in distance running

Henrik Larsen

Synopsis

This chapter reviews the significance of intensity, frequency, duration and volume of training on performance and physiological adaptations to endurance training with special emphasis on distance running. The role of each of these factors is described primarily on the basis of knowledge derived from scientific training studies performed on initially untrained subjects but also from training studies exploring well-trained subjects including elite athletes. Furthermore, based on some case studies linkage is made between knowledge derived from studies of training performed by elite runners and knowledge derived from science.

Introduction

Over the last several decades many attempts have been made to elucidate the exact nature of the endurance-training stimulus and the most efficient procedure by which it may be elicited. The question as to what is the optimal stimulus for adaptation to endurance training including long-distance running and with that improved performance has constantly challenged researchers. Intensive research has led to a better understanding of the different factors of importance for optimal improvement although many questions still remains unsolved.

Crucial factors determining success in middle- and long distance running events include the functional capacity of the cardiovascular system, the capacity for aerobic and anaerobic energy turnover, muscular strength, running economy, skeletal muscle fibre composition, mitochondrial oxidative capacity, motivation and tactics. Outstanding performance in long distance running primarily requires an optimal combination of high maximal aerobic power, good running economy and a high fractional utilisation of $\dot{V}O_2$-max during competition. The significance of these factors have been expressed in the following equation by di Prampero and collaborators (9):

$$vEND = \frac{F \cdot \dot{V}O_2\text{-max}}{C}$$

where vEND is the maximal speed sustainable during endurance running, F the maximal fraction of $\dot{V}O_2$-max that can be maintained throughout the duration of the effort in question, and C the energy spent per unit distance. Capelli & di Prampero (see page 67) and Svedenhag (see page 85) carefully describes the significance of C (running economy). Therefore, an essential focus in the present chapter is on crucial physiological variables required for reaching and maintaining a high maximal energy turnover, and to describe how these variables adapt to training.

Many physiological variables have been identified as important for transport of oxygen from the atmosphere to the working muscles and thus for energy production.

The *lung diffusion capacity* is not considered to be a primary limiting factor for $\dot{V}O_2$-max except in well-trained elite athletes (8).

Cardiac output is determined by heart rate multiplied by stroke volume. Heart volume is essential for stroke volume and thus minute volume, which in turn has been shown to be a major determinant of $\dot{V}O_2$-max. A lowered heart rate at a constant work rate caused by endurance training is a classical finding within the scientific physiological literature.

Blood volume and particularly the total volume of haemoglobin has been shown to be of major importance for $\dot{V}O_2$-max (e.g. 11). Additionally, $\dot{V}O_2$-max depends on the arteriovenous oxygen difference.

Capillarisation is one of the factors determining the oxidative profile of the musculature. The capillary density has been shown to correlate positively with the running velocity at which blood lactate begins to accumulate (49), which in turn has been found to correlate with running velocity during competitions of various distances (e.g. 14).

The activity of *oxidative enzymes* in the muscles has been shown to be essential for the respiratory capacity of the muscle tissue (23). This has in turn been shown to be significantly related to the level of blood lactate at given work rates (27). This implies, that running speed at a given blood lactate level as well as oxygen uptake per minute per kg of body weight at a given blood lactate level is highly related to performance in running.

Adaptations to training of the enumerated physiological variables have been investigated in numerous scientific investigations. Most of these variables have been shown to be dependent upon the training stimulus and the training principles.

In the present chapter the role of some of the most important factors for reaching an optimal physiological training stimulus will be presented with the main focus on distance running. However when suitable research derived from other endurance sports and general endurance exercise will be included. Additionally some case studies will be presented. Important factors to be highlighted are training intensity, frequency, duration and volume.

Training intensity

The significance of training intensity has been studied extensively but although an optimal intensity has not yet been identified it is almost generally accepted that the intensity is of great importance for the training response. Numerous studies performed at training intensities between 36 and 170% of $\dot{V}O_2$-max have shown a positive training response.

Training threshold

Several studies have noted the existence of a training threshold, in terms of intensity, below which no training response is seen. This minimal stimulus necessary to evoke training adaptations has been reported to be at about 50% of $\dot{V}O_2$-max (6), 75% of maximal heart rate (2), slightly above the 60% training level (max. heart rate-resting heart rate) (28) or a heart rate of 140-150 beats $\cdot$ min^{-1} (13, 53). Indeed one study performed at intensities from 35 to 55% of $\dot{V}O_2$-max in subjects previously training 3 x 45 min • week^{-1} showed no additional training effect at all, even if the subjects exercised 5.5 hours • day^{-1}, 6 days • week^{-1} for 8 weeks (45). However, in a study by Nordesjö (39) adaptation to training was observed after exercise at 36% of $\dot{V}O_2$-max while other investigations have shown adaptations after training at 45% of $\dot{V}O_2$-max (19, 24). In addition, it has been suggested that adaptation to training can occur at exercise intensity producing a heart rate of 110-120 beats • min^{-1} in sedentary population with low levels of habitual activity (48). The difficulty of identifying the lower limit of adaptation to training may be due to the fact that many studies have shown that the training response is dependent upon the initial physical condition of the individual (e.g. 44, 57).

Significance of exercise above the training threshold

Several studies on previously untrained subjects have shown that a higher training response measured either by work capacity (39), work capacity and $\dot{V}O_2$-max (57), $\dot{V}O_2$-max (48), $\dot{V}O_2$-max and oxygen consumption at fixed blood lactate concentrations (56), $\dot{V}O_2$ at lactate threshold (24) or arteriovenous oxygen difference (32) is achieved in subjects training at the highest intensities. Other investigations have shown identical training response in subjects training at different intensities above the training threshold (2, 19, 21, 47, 53). However the lack of difference in training response in some of these studies may be due to the fact that some of them were performed with a limited training period (10 days to 6 weeks). One study demonstrated that the length of the study period is critical for significant adaptations to occur (41). In this investigation no differences in cardiorespiratory response to training were observed between groups jogging either 2 or 4 days • week^{-1} after 10 weeks. However significant differences in several variables were seen after completing 20 weeks of training. A few studies comparing groups training at different intensities and quantities have demonstrated that the same improvement in either performance and activities of hexokinase, phosphorylase, phosphofructokinase, succinate dehydrogenase, and 3-hydroxyacyl CoA dehydrogenase enzymes (26), $\dot{V}O_2$-max (43) or submaximal heart rate/$\dot{V}O_2$-max (17) can be achieved when training at higher intensities but smaller quantities. Equal improvements in $\dot{V}O_2$-max were also seen in a study comparing training

5 hours • week^{-1} at 70% of $\dot{V}O_2$-max with very short (20 s) high-intensity intermittent training sessions performed at 170% of $\dot{V}O_2$-max (55). In addition, this latter study showed a significant increase in anaerobic capacity in the high intensity-training group. Furthermore a detraining study examining the effect of a reduction in training intensity, while maintaining training frequency and duration, showed losses in $\dot{V}O_2$-max, left ventricular mass and endurance performance within 5 to 15 weeks (25).

Effect of adding short intensive training to moderate training

Six studies on well-trained athletes have demonstrated increased training responses when short intensive training sessions either were added or partly/fully replaced the normal training at moderate intensity. Thus, adding one intensive 20 min treadmill run • week^{-1} to the normal 5.7 hours of running • week^{-1} at low intensity resulted in an increase in running speed eliciting a blood lactate concentration of 4 mmol • l^{-1} (50). In addition high intensity (90-95% of $\dot{V}O_2$-max) interval training (3 d • week^{-1}) improved both 10-km race performance and exercise time to fatigue at supramaximal running speed and decreased plasma lactate concentration at 85 and 90% of $\dot{V}O_2$-max in competitive runners (1). In another study replacing 82 km • week^{-1} of running at moderate intensity with high intensity running and cycling 6 d • week^{-1} (40 min running, HR of ~ 190 beats • min^{-1}, 3 days • week^{-1} and 5 x 5 min on cycle ergometer, HR of ~ 180, 3 days • week^{-1}) improved the 10-km run time despite of a marked decrease in training volume (35). Furthermore replacing 15% of the normal 300 km • week^{-1} of endurance cycle training with high-intensity interval training in three different studies increased the peak power output and the 40-km time-trial performance (30, 58, 59). Moreover, in two of these investigations an enhancement of the "anaerobic performance" (time to fatigue at 150% of peak power output) was observed (30, 59) along with an increase in skeletal muscle buffering capacity in one of these studies (59). Additionally, the study by Westgart-Taylor and collaborators (58) demonstrated decreases in carbohydrate oxidation, plasma lactate concentration and ventilation when the cyclists rode at the same absolute work rates of 60, 70 and 80% of initial peak power output after completion of the high intensity training period.

Response to increased training intensity
of entire training performed

Two studies have examined the physiological response to an increase in training intensity of all the training performed. One study in which normal training of 2.2 h • week^{-1} with a mean training intensity of 65% of maximum heart rate (HR$_{max}$) was increased to 2.7 h • week^{-1} and an average intensity of 78% of HR$_{max}$ revealed significant increases in $\dot{V}O_2$-max and exercise time to exhaustion at 86% of pre-training $\dot{V}O_2$-max (31). It is true that at least some of the improvement may be due to the fact that the training volume was increased, but since even a large training volume increase has shown relatively minor improvement of performance time (4) the increase in performance time (74%) in the present study cannot be explained by an elevation of training volume alone. This view is supported by cross-sectional studies investigating performance and training volume (e.g. 16, 33). Another study comparing two groups of elite junior cross-country skiers who trained at either moderate intensity (60-70% of $\dot{V}O_2$-max) or high intensity (80-90% of $\dot{V}O_2$-max), 12-15 hours • week^{-1} for 5 months, showed a more profound training response (performance in a 20-min run test) in the high, than in the moderate intensity training group (12). Additionally, the activity of the mitochondrial enzyme succinate dehydrogenase (SDH) rose by 6% and the phosphofructokinase (PFK) activity fell by 10% in the high intensity-training group, while no changes were observed in the group training at moderate intensity. Furthermore, positive correlations between the activity of CS, SDH and GPHD enzymes and performance were found.

In a study of elite runners in and off-season, a small but significant enhancement in $\dot{V}O_2$-max was observed in season compared to off-season. This change seemed to be due to the higher training intensity performed during the preparation period prior to the competitive season (54). Moreover a minor but significant improvement in running economy was found in this study during one year of continuous training.

Athletes studied during three successive summer training periods

In a study by Rusko (42), performed on young cross-country skiers during a three-year period, two different groups of skiers were compared. One group trained at a relatively low total training volume, but with a relatively high volume and frequency of interval type training performed at high intensity, while another group trained at a relatively large total training volume but with a relatively small volume of intensive training. The study revealed that training at high intensity/low total volume resulted in a significant increase in $\dot{V}O_2$-max, while no change was seen after training at low intensity, despite the fact that a significantly greater total training volume was performed.

Cross-sectional studies

Two cross-sectional studies performed on marathon runners examining the relationship between marathon performance and various training components revealed a significant correlation between average training pace (intensity) and performance (22, 38). In line with this, Foster (16) investigated the relationship between performance in 1.0; 2.0; 3.0; 6.0; 10.0 and 26.2 mile races and training intensity in another cross-sectional study and found significant correlations between training speed and performance in the different distances. The correlations were not strong, and the strength of the correlations tended to decrease as the competition distance decreased. However these large-scale correlate studies do support the importance of training intensity.

Training at the individual anaerobic threshold

It has been hypothesised that training at the individual lactate threshold often named anaerobic threshold is beneficial for the training response (e.g. 50). This threshold has been defined either as the intensity eliciting a given concentration of lactate in the venous blood (e.g. 4 mmol • l^{-1}) or the intensity where a non-linear increase in lactate concentration is observed. However, an investigation comparing groups training either 30 min at the individual anaerobic threshold (IAT) or four times 7.5

min at intensities which alternated between being below (IAT – 30 % of the difference between $\dot{V}O_2$-max and IAT) and above the IAT (IAT + 30 % of the difference between $\dot{V}O_2$-max and IAT) demonstrated no differences in physiological adaptations between groups (29). In addition to the finding that training at IAT does not seem to be crucial, the study indicates that the physiological adaptations are independent of whether the exercise is performed intermittently or continuously. It is true that exercising at IAT (4 mmol • l^{-1}) is effective (50). However, this is not surprising since a relatively high training intensity is crucial for the training response. Based on the investigations described above (12, 31, 56) training at IAT – 30 % of the difference between $\dot{V}O_2$-max and IAT is hardly an effective training intensity because the stimulus probably is too low. Since identical adaptations were observed in the two training groups exercising either at or above/below IAT, it can be argued that training at IAT + 30 % of the difference between $\dot{V}O_2$-max and IAT is advantageous compared to training at IAT. It is obvious to conclude that there is no scientific evidence that exercise at IAT is the optimal training intensity. Furthermore, the scientific literature on this topic has revealed that it is difficult to identify IAT and to perform training exactly at IAT (50). In addition the term "anaerobic threshold" is misleading because lactate is normally produced under fully aerobic conditions in the muscle. Moreover, training at IAT cannot be recommended because it causes a lot of practical implications.

Training frequency

Frequency of endurance training defined as the number of training bouts during a given time has been shown to be important determinants for improving various physiological functions and performance.

Four different kind of study design has been used in order to investigate training frequency.

1. Investigations examining the effect of increased number of training sessions • $week^{-1}$ with a fixed duration of each single bout, thereby reflecting increased training volume.
2. Cross-sectional studies.
3. Studies exploring training frequency with a fixed training volume.
4. Investigations examining the timing of the training sessions during the training week.

Studies examining training frequency and increased training volume

The vast majority of studies have focused on the role of the weekly number of training bouts performed with a fixed duration of each bout and the existence of a direct relationship between frequency of training and the adaptation of different physiological variables and performance is almost generally accepted. Some of these studies have shown that the improvement of $\dot{V}O_2$-max increases in proportion to frequency of training (6, 20, 40, 41, 48). Likewise, improvement of work capacity/performance has been shown to occur in proportion to training frequency (20, 39). Additionally, some studies have shown reduction in body weight and percent body fat (40), total body and fat weight (41) and reduction in percent body fat (20) in groups training 4-5 times • week[-1] compared to groups training 2 times • week[-1]. Moreover, training 4 times • week[-1] compared to 2 times • week[-1] has shown superior improvements in $\dot{V}O_2$-max and submaximal HR during a standard treadmill run, as well a more rapid decrease in HR during recovery and a lower resting HR (20, 41). Although significantly higher physiological adaptations were registered in the group training with the highest frequency in the study by Pollock and colleagues (40) no difference were observed between groups in a 2-mile run.

In one study comparing the training response in groups performing interval run training either 2 or 4 times per week for 7 and 13 weeks, respectively, no differences in elevation of $\dot{V}O_2$-max were observed (18). However the lack of difference in response between groups may be due to the fact that the $\dot{V}O_2$-max-tests were performed on bicycle ergometer, which do not fully reflect changes in running $\dot{V}O_2$-max. Even though the enhancement of $\dot{V}O_2$-max was identical between groups, different adaptations in submaximal heart rates measured during work loads demanding 80-85% of $\dot{V}O_2$-max was registered.

Thus the decrease in heart rate was significantly greater in the 4 days • week[-1] groups than in the 2 days • week[-1] groups for both the 7- and 13-week training programs. In addition, the decrease in submaximal heart rate was significantly greater in the group training twice per week for 13 weeks compared to the group training twice per week for 7 weeks. However, no differences were observed between groups training 4 days • week[-1] for 7 or 13 weeks.

Cross-sectional studies

The notion that training frequency is important for the training response is supported by a cross-sectional study performed by Hagan and colleagues (22) on marathon runners. In this investigation the total number of training sessions in the preparation period (9 weeks) prior to a marathon race showed to be very important for the performance time. Thus, a highly significant correlation of −0.62 between training frequency and marathon time was found. This is in agreement with the findings by Marti and collaborators (33), who showed a significant association between 16-km running time and weekly training frequency.

Studies examining frequency with a fixed training volume

One very relevant question that arises concerning the above mentioned investigations, is the degree to which the observed physiological adaptations is the result of an increased number of training bouts per se, or rather that training frequency results in a proportional increase in training volume.

A few studies have evaluated the effect of training with different training frequencies but kept the weekly training volume at a fixed level (7, 37). This design implies that the duration of the single training bout varies in direct proportion to the weekly number of training bouts. Thus, these studies evaluate the effect of the number of training sessions and the role of the duration of each single training session at the same time. In one study using this design one group jogged 30 min • day^{-1} at 65-75% of peak heart rate while another group completed three 10-min jogging bouts daily at the same training intensity separated by at least 4 hours (7). The training caused a significant increase in maximal oxygen uptake in both training groups but the increase was significantly greater in the group training continuous 30 min • day^{-1}. However, the increase in exercise test duration as well as the decrease in heart rate at submaximal exercise was similar in both groups. In another study using the same kind of design two groups of women completed either three 10-min training bouts or one 30-min bout per day, 5 days • week^{-1} for 10 weeks (37). The training consisted of brisk walking at 70 to 80% of maximal heart rate. The training resulted in significant increases in $\dot{V}O_2$-max and $\dot{V}O_2$ at blood lactate concentration of 2 mmol • l^{-1} in both training groups but no differences were observed between groups. The view that the response to training is independent of training frequency and thus duration if the training volume is fixed gets support by a study from Marti and collaborators (33).

These researchers compared 414 runners all taking part in a 16 km competition who had the same training background in terms of training volume (20-25 km • week^{-1}), but who had achieved this volume by performing either 2, 3 or 4 training sessions • week^{-1}. Despite the considerable difference in training frequency and duration of the single training bout no significant differences in performance were observed.

Placement of training bouts during the week

One study using a different design was undertaken in order to investigate the effect of "placement" of training sessions during the week (36). In this study one group of subjects performed high intensity type running (five 3-min exercise bouts) on Monday, Tuesday, and Wednesday for 10 weeks. Another group of subjects performed a similar training protocol with the exception that training sessions were conducted on Monday, Wednesday, and Friday. Both groups improved $\dot{V}O_2$-max significantly following the ten weeks of training. In addition the heart rate at a given submaximal workload was lowered significantly in both groups. However no significant physiological differences were found between the groups. Even if all tests were performed on a bicycle ergometer the results indicate that a specific placement of tri-weekly training sessions of running is not critical with respect to enhancement of aerobic capacity.

Training duration

Numerous studies have shown that duration of the single training session is an important stimulus for eliciting a training response. Increased training duration has resulted in significant improvement in $\dot{V}O_2$-max (6, 48), work capacity (39), cardiovascular capacity/work capacity (60) and $\dot{V}O_2$-max/performance (34). However, training duration does not in itself seem to stimulate the training response. As mentioned earlier, the study performed at intensities from 35 to 55% of $\dot{V}O_2$-max on moderately trained subjects showed no training effect at all, even if the subjects exercised 5.5 hours per day, 6 days per week for 8 weeks (45).

Cross-sectional studies

The studies mentioned earlier (22, 38) performed on marathon runners during the preparation period prior to a marathon race supports the view that distance/duration of the single training bout is important for the training response. Thus, Hagan and collaborators (22) found a significant correlation between marathon performance time and average km • workout[1]. In addition, Murray and colleagues (38) showed a significant correlation between the number of training runs longer than 15 miles and performance in marathon.

As described in regards to training frequency the same kind of question arises concerning some of the above-enumerated investigations. To what extend are the observed physiological adaptations due to the increased training duration per se or by the fact that training volume increases in direct proportion to training duration? The three studies mentioned earlier (7, 33, 37) comparing different groups training with identical weekly training volume but with different training frequency/duration show that training duration is not of any major importance for the training response. However, one of these studies indicates that duration may be important for the increase in $\dot{V}O_2$-max (7).

Two studies having compared training programs keeping the total work amount at a constant level have shown that a higher $\dot{V}O_2$-max and increased work capacity can be achieved if the training is performed at high intensity and short duration of the single training session (57) or that identical improvements in $\dot{V}O_2$-max can be achieved using a shorter duration of the single training bout performed with higher training intensity (47).

Training volume

Surveys through the scientific literature reveal that training volume is essential for the training response and the adaptations of numerous physiological variables. This is well in line with the view taken by coaches and runners, and often carried to extremes. The view that training volume is of major significance at least up to a certain upper limit, is true. Whether there exists an upper ceiling for adaptation to training, is not known, but likely depends on the adaptive potential of the individual athlete.

The majority of physiological investigations examining training volume are made on marathon running and without exception these studies have shown training volume to be of major importance for success at this distance. In addition, the training volume in the last two months preceding the event appears to be an essential part of the preparation for the race (10, 15, 16, 22, 38, 49, 51, 52). Furthermore, not only the training volume during the last two months prior to the competition, but the volume of the total distance covered during the last year before the marathon, has been shown to be of equally great importance (10). However almost all investigations concerning marathon performance have been based on cross-sectional samples, and may presumably be confounded by the tendency for runners having the right genetic "make up" to train harder and perform higher training volume than less talented runners. In addition high correlations are to be expected in studies of runners with very wide ranges of performance capacities. Therefore, the significance of the observed relationship between training volume and performance is difficult to evaluate. However, in one study examining the effect of an increase in training volume from 76 to 91 km • week^{-1} (20%), experienced runners improved marathon performance time significantly from 3 h 20.7 min to 3 h 10.8 min (5%) (15).

The investigation mentioned above by Foster (16) demonstrated not only a significant relationship between marathon performance and training volume, but also significant correlations between training volume and performance in 1, 2, 3, 6 and 10 miles races were revealed.

In agreement with this, Marti and colleagues (33) demonstrated that the weekly training distance calculated during the last year prior to the competition was significantly associated to performance in a 16 km-run. Moreover, this investigation showed that the regression line reflecting the mean relation between habitual mileage and running time is not linear but levels off in the range of 80 to 100 km • week^{-1}. This observation is in line with observations by Costill (3) in an investigation of two runners, who following a six-month layoff gradually increased their weekly mileage. $\dot{V}O_2$-max increased when the mileage increased to 50 and also 75 miles • week^{-1}. Beyond that level no additional gains in $\dot{V}O_2$-max were seen, even if the subjects continued training and reached 225 miles • week^{-1} on the average during a one-month period.

In addition to the above-enumerated investigations studying relationship between training volume and marathon performance in large groups of runners with a wide range of performance capacities, Sjödin & Svedenhag (51) examined the same relationship within 3 different categories of runners. The subgroups consisted of elite runners with personal record (PR) below 2 hour 30 minutes, good runners with PR between 2 hours 30 minutes and 3 hours and slow runners with PR above 3 hours. The average weekly number of kilometres of these runners were 57, 115 and 145 km • week^{-1}, respectively, and significant correlation's between training volume and performance were found within each of these subgroups. In addition, significant differences in $\dot{V}O_2$-max were observed between all three subgroups. The percentage of $\dot{V}O_2$-max utilised during the marathon was also found to be significantly lower in the group performing the lowest weekly training volume compared to the two other training groups. No difference in % of $\dot{V}O_2$-max was observed between the two groups running 115 and 145 km • week^{-1}, respectively. Therefore the authors speculate, whether there may be an upper limit of training distance, above which there is no further increase in the percentage of $\dot{V}O_2$-max sustained during a marathon race. However, the authors suggest that a huge training volume may shorten the recovery period after races and may preserve good form for subsequent performances.

Another reason for performing high training volume may be that the higher training volume improves running economy which has been suggested by Scrimgeour and colleagues (46) in a cross-sectional study, and which is in line with Daniels (5) and colleagues who have suggested that a certain threshold of training may be needed for inducing a significant change in running economy. In the study by Scrimgeour and colleagues (46) three groups of runners, competing in various racing distances from 10 to 90 km and training either less than 60 km • week^{-1}, 60-100 km • week^{-1} or more than 100 km • week^{-1} were compared. The results showed that runners training more than 100 km • week^{-1} had significantly faster running times at all distances (average 19,2%) than those with less than 100 km • week^{-1}. Additionally, the study revealed that neither $\dot{V}O_2$-max nor %$\dot{V}O_2$-max sustained during competition was different between groups. On the other hand, the findings showed that the faster speed of the more trained runners was due to superior running economy (20%). Therefore, the group differences could be explained on the basis of differences in running economy alone, which suggests that the main effect of training more than 100 km • week^{-1} may be an improvement of running economy, or alternatively that runners training more than 100 km • week^{-1} may have superior running economy due to genetic reasons.

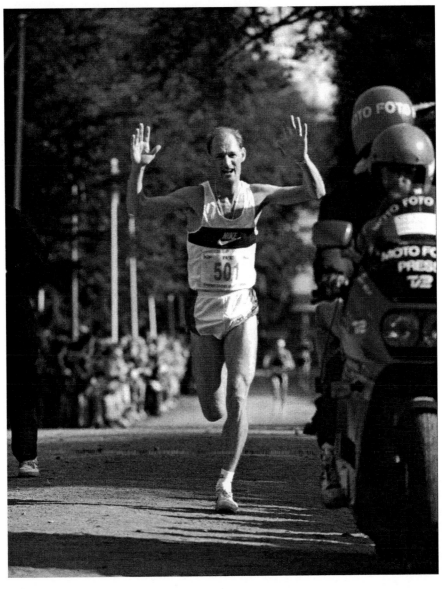

Case studies

There seems to be a close relationship between knowledge derived from scientific investigations and knowledge based on selected case studies of training performed by elite runners. In order to demonstrate this specific relationship three case studies will be presented. Elite runners who have all used different training methods and changed their training strategy radically during their career are selected. Studies of these runners reveal a unique possibility to compare the impact of the different training principles. Characteristic years representing different training principles are highlighted. The described data are primarily derived from studies of training logbooks but also from personal communication.

Flemming Jensen (FJ) Danish record holder in 3000 m steeplechase

1978-1980
The training performed by FJ was sparse and not well organised. He trained for and competed in various distances on track during the summer and practised orienteering during the winter. During 1980 the training volume exceeded 100 km • week^{-1}.

1981
During the preparation period (17 weeks) the average weekly training performed encompassed the following:
Training: *Volume:* 160 km • week^{-1}
         Intensity of 150 km • week^{-1}: 4 min • km^{-1}
         Interval: 10 km • week^{-1}, (e.g. 10 x 400 m, 1 min rest between repetitions)
         One weekly training session longer than 20 km
Based on this training, FJ achieved the following results:
         3000 m steeplechase: 8 min 56 s
         10000 m: 29 min 55 s
         15 km: 46 min 35 s

1983

FJ changed his training radically. The total training volume was decreased, while the average intensity was increased considerably. Moreover, the volume of intervals was increased and longer intervals were introduced because of the probable positive effect on $\dot{V}O_2$-max of these intervals. There was a complete lack of this kind of interval training in 1981.

During the preparation period (17 weeks) the average weekly training performed encompassed the following:

Training: *Volume:* 100 km • week^{-1}

Intensity of 85 km • week^{-1}: 3 min 35 s • km^{-1}

Interval training: 15 km • week^{-1}, (e.g. 6 x 1000 m or 3 x 1000 m, 3 x 600 m, 3 x 400 m, with 3 min rest between all repetitions)

No training sessions longer than 15 km

On the basis of this training, the following results were achieved:

3000 m steeplechase: 8 min 31 s

5000 m: 14 min 19 s

10000 m: 29 min 45 s

15 km: 47 min 25 s

It appears that the steeplechase time improved significantly, while the 15-km time decreased slightly.

1987

The total training volume was enhanced slightly, but was still below the magnitude achieved in 1981. The average intensity was also further increased while the interval training was unchanged, compared to what was performed in 1983.

Training: *Volume:* 120 km • week^{-1}

Intensity of the entire training performed: 3 min 17 s • km^{-1}

Interval training: 15 km • week^{-1}, (e.g. 3 x 1000 m, 3 x 600 m and 3 x 400 m, 3 min rest or 6 x 1000 m, 3 min rest between repetitions)

No sessions longer than 15 km

After performing this training, FJ achieved the following results:

3000 m steeplechase: 8 min 23 s

5000 m: 13 min 36 s

10-km road race: 28 min 46 s

15 km: 44 min 45 s

The above enumerated data supports the view that training intensity is of great importance, not only when it comes to intensity and volume of interval training, but also – the intensity of the distance training performed between the interval-days seems to be crucial, at least as long as the total training volume is relatively small. It is true that the training volume performed by FJ was sparse prior to 1981 and that it probably takes years of hard training to approach the upper limit of adaptation to training. Therefore it can be argued that FJ probably would have improved performance after 1981 even without the described change in training principles. However, improved performance results achieved by FJ due to an increased training intensity is very much in agreement with findings from several scientific studies (e.g. 1, 12, 56).

Henrik Jørgensen (HJ) – Scandinavian record holder in marathon and winner of the London Marathon (1988)

1978-1985
HJ based his training primarily on long, relatively slow ($\sim$4 min 5 s $\cdot$ km^{-1}) distance runs. In addition he performed various forms of interval training. The total average weekly training distance during these years was 164 (range 129-185) km $\cdot$ week^{-1}. Included in this training HJ performed various kind of interval training, which averaged 13.3 (9.6 -16.2) km $\cdot$ week^{-1}.

1985
During the last 16 weeks prior to the London Marathon, the average weekly training performed encompassed the following:

Training: *Volume:* 205 km $\cdot$ week^{-1}
Frequency: 13 sessions $\cdot$ week^{-1}
Intensity of 193 km: 4 min $\cdot$ km^{-1}
Interval: 12 km $\cdot$ week^{-1}, $<$ 3 min $\cdot$ km^{-1}
One weekly session longer than 24 km

Based on this training Henrik finished third in the London Marathon in 2 h 9 min 43 s.

1986-87

HJ continued training using the same concept without achieving any remarkable results. After failing in the London Marathon in 1987, HJ changed his training to a large extent. Both the speed of his distance runs and the volume of interval training increased considerably.

During the last 12 weeks prior to the world championships in Rome (1987) the average week had the following content:

Training: *Volume:* 167 (152-182) km • week^{-1}

Frequency: 15 (13-16) sessions • week^{-1}

Intensity of the entire training performed: 3 min 23 s (3:20-3:26) • km^{-1}.

Interval: 23 km • week^{-1} ($<$ 3 min • km^{-1}) (e.g. 4 x 2 km or 3 x 4 km)

No sessions longer than 15 km

After performing this kind of training Henrik finished 9th in marathon at the world championships. Due to very high temperatures for marathon running the finishing time was 2 h 14 min 58 s.

1987-88

After a couple of weeks without training due to illness HJ started training for the London Marathon 1988. He tried to continue training in the same way, but failed to reach the intended volume.

The content of the average weekly training during the last 14 weeks prior to the London Marathon is described below:

Training: *Volume:* 136 (115-170) km • week^{-1}

Frequency: 14 (13-16) sessions • week^{-1}

Intensity of the entire training performed: 3 min 29 s (3:26-3:31) • km^{-1}

Interval: 13 km • week^{-1}, $<$ 3 min • km^{-1} (e.g. 4 x 2 km; 3 x 4 km)

No sessions longer than 15 km

Rather surprisingly, based on this training HJ won the London Marathon. Despite bad weather conditions and the fact that HJ was running the last 7 km alone he won in 2 h 10 min 20 s. The above described training and results seem to confirm the findings described in different scientific papers (e.g. 39), namely that the same work capacity (performance) can be achieved after completion of a relatively small training volume performed at high intensity instead of performing a great training volume at a relatively low intensity.

Gert Kærlin (GK) – Danish record holder in 5000 m (1973-1982)

In contrast to the change in training principles described above for HJ and FJ, respectively, the training performed by GK changed from a relatively small volume with high intensity to a considerably greater training volume with relatively low intensity during the preparation period for competition. During many years before 1976, GK based his training on a relatively small training volume during the winter and an even smaller training volume during the summer. In addition, various intervals of high intensity were performed each second day during the summer period.

1973

A typical training week during the preparation period consisted of the following:

Training: *Volume:* 110 km • week⁻¹

Frequency: 7-9 sessions • week⁻¹

Intensity: Not exactly known

Interval: 2 times • week⁻¹ (e.g. 20 x 400 m, ~1 min rest between repetitions or 6 x 1000 m, 2 min rest between repetitions).

No sessions longer than 18 km

Based on this training GK improved the Danish record in 5000 m by running 13 min 40 s.

The same kind of training as described above continued until the winter 1975/76. During this period the total volume increased considerably, while the training intensity decreased.

1976

A typical training week included the following:

Training: *Volume:* 200 km • week⁻¹

Frequency: 10-11 sessions • week⁻¹

Intensity: Not exactly known

Interval: Mainly anaerobic of "fartlek"-type

At least two weekly sessions longer than 22 km

After performing this kind of training GK broke his own Danish record in 5000 m by running 13 min 39 s but since the improvement was extremely small, it is obvious to conclude, that the same performance level can be achieved after completion of a relatively small training volume performed at high intensity compared to a great training volume performed at a relatively low intensity.

Additionally, the training performed and the results achieved by HJ and GK indicate that the same performance level is reached regardless of whether a large total training volume performed at relatively low intensities is exchanged with a relatively smaller total training volume performed at relatively high intensities, or that these different training programs are performed in reverse order.

Furthermore, since both HJ and GK seem to have reached or have been very close to an upper limit of adaptation to training, the presented case studies support the view that there exists an upper limit beyond which no adaptation to training take place.

Concluding remarks

- The intensity of training is of extreme significance for physiological adaptations as well as performance.
- Training frequency and duration of a single training session are important for the training response, if an increase of these factors implies increased training volume. However, evidence that training frequency vs. training duration is of any significance if the training volume is fixed is weak.
- Training volume is essential for physiological adaptations and performance. Whether there may be an upper training limit beyond which no improvement in physiological adaptations and performance is seen with increased training is still not clear, but it is likely to depend on the individual's capacity to adapt as well as to tolerate varying volumes of high intensity training.

References

1. Acevedo, E.O. and Goldfarb, A.H. Increased training intensity effects on plasma lactate, ventilatory threshold, and endurance. *Med Sci Sports Exerc,* 21(5), 563-568, 1989.
2. Burke, E.J. and Franks, B.D. Changes in $\dot{V}O_2$-max resulting from bicycle training at different intensities holding total mechanical work constant. *Res Q,* 46, 31-37, 1975.

3. Costill, D.L. Training: The Price for Success. In: *Inside Running: Basics of sports physiology.* Benchmark Press, Inc. ISBN: 0-93615700-3, 85-121, 1986.

4. Daniels, J.T., Yarbrough, R.A. and Foster, C. Changes in VO_2-max and running performance with training. *Eur J Appl Physiol,* 39, 249-254, 1978.

5. Daniels, J.T. A physiologist's view of running economy. *Med Sci Sports Exerc,* 17, 332-338, 1985.

6. Davies, C.T.M. and Knibbs, A.V. The training stimulus: the effects of intensity, duration and frequency of effort on maximum aerobic power output. *Int Z Angew,* 29, 299-305, 1971.

7. DeBusk, R.F., Stenestrand, U., Sheehan, M. and Haskell, W.L. Training effects of long versus short bouts of exercise in healthy subjects. *Am J Cardiol,* 65, 1010-1013, 1990.

8. Dempsey, J.A., Hansson, P.G. and Henderson, K.S. Exercise-induced arterial hypoxaemia in healthy human subjects at sea level. *J Physiol,* 355, 161-175, 1984.

9. di Prampero, P.E., Atchou, G., Brückner, J.-C. and Moia, C. The energetics of endurance running. *Eur J Appl Physiol,* 55, 259-266, 1986.

10. Dotan, R., Rotstein, R., Dlin, R., Inbar, O., Kofman, H. and Kaplansky, Y. Relationships of marathon running to physiological, anthropometric and training indices. *Eur J Appl Physiol,* 51, 281-293, 1983.

11. Ekblom, B., Goldbarg, A.N. and Gullbring, B. Response to exercise after blood loss and reinfusion. *J Appl Physiol,* 33(2), 175-80, 1972.

12. Evertsen, F., Medbo, J.I., Jebens, E. and Gjovaag, T.F. Effect of training on the activity of five muscle enzymes studied on elite cross-country skiers. *Acta Physiol Scand,* 167(3), 247-57, 1999.

13. Faria, E.F. Cardiovascular response to exercise as influenced by training of various intensities. *Res Q,* 41(1), 44-50, 1970.

14. Farrell, P.A., Wilmore, J.H., Coyle, E.F., Billing, J.E. and Costill, D.L. Plasma lactate accumulation and distance running performance. *Med Sci Sports,* 11(4), 338-344, 1979.

15. Foster, C., Daniels, J.T. and Yarbrough, R.A. Physiological and training correlates of marathon running performance. *Aust J Sports Med,* 9, 58-61, 1977.

16. Foster, C. VO_2-max and training indices as determinants of competitive running performance. *J Sports Sci,* 1, 13-22, 1983.

17. Fox, E.L., Bartels, R.L., Billings, C.E., Mathews, D.K., Bason, R. and Webb, W.M. Intensity and distance of interval training programs and change in aerobic power. *Med Sci Sports,* 5(1), 18-22, 1973.

18. Fox, E.L., Bartels, R.L., Billings, C.E., O'brian, R., Bason, R. and Mathews, D.K. Frequency and duration of interval training programs and change in aerobic power. *J Appl Physiol,* 38(3), 481-484, 1975.

19. Gaesser, G.A. and Rich, R.G. Effects of high- and low- intensity exercise training on aerobic capacity and blood lipids. *Med Sci Sports Exerc,* 16(3), 269-274, 1984.

20. Gettman, L.R., Pollock, M.L., Durstine, J.L., Ward, A., Ayres, J. and Linnerud, A.C. Physiological responses of men to 1, 3, and 5 day per week training programs. *Res Q,* 47(4), 638-646, 1976.

21. Gregory, L.W. The development of aerobic capacity: A comparison of continuous and interval training. *Res Q,* 50(2), 199-206, 1979.

22. Hagan, R.D., Smith, M.G. and Gettman, L.R. Marathon performance in relation to maximal aerobic power and training indices. *Med Sci Sports Exerc,* 13(3), 185-189, 1981.

23. Henriksson, J. Training induced adaptation of skeletal muscle and metabolism during submaximal exercise. *J Physiol (Lond),* 270(3), 661-75, 1977.

24. Henritze, J., Weltman, A., Schurrer, R.L. and Barlow, K. Effects of training at and above the lactate threshold on the lactate threshold and maximal oxygen uptake. *Eur J Appl Physiol,* 54, 84-88, 1985.

25. Hickson, R.C., Foster, C., Pollock, M.L., Galassi, T.M. and Rich, S. Reduced training intensities and loss of aerobic power, endurance and cardiac growth. *J Appl Physiol,* 58(2), 492-499, 1985.

26. Houston, M.E., Wilson, D.M., Green, H.J., Thomson, J.A. and Ranney, D.A. Physiological and muscle enzyme adaptations to different intensities of swim training. *Eur J Appl Physiol,* 46, 283-291, 1981.

27. Ivy, J.L., Withers, R.T., van Handel, P.J., Elger, D.H. and Costill, D.L. Muscle respiratory capacity and fiber type as determinants of the lactate threshold. *J Appl Physiol: Respirat. Environ. Exercise Physiol,* 48(3), 523-527, 1980.

28. Karvonen, M.J., Kentala, E. and Mustala, O. The effects of training on heart rate. A "longitudinal" study. *Ann Med Exper Biol Fenn* 35, 307-315, 1957.

29. Keith, S.P., Jacobs, I. and McLellan, T.M. Adaptations to training at the individual anaerobic threshold. *Eur J Appl Physiol,* 65, 316-323, 1992.

30. Lindsay, F.H., Hawley, J.A., Myburgh, K.H., Schomer, H.H., Noakes, T.D., Dennis, S.C. Improved athletic performance in highly trained cyclists after interval training. *Med Sci Sports Exer,* 28(11), 1427-1434, 1996.

31. Madsen, K., Franch, J. and Clausen, T. Effects of intensified endurance training on the concentration of Na, K-ATPase and Ca-ATPase in human skeletal muscle. *Acta Physiol Scand,* 150, 251-258, 1994.

32. Massicotte, D.R. and Avon, G. Cardiovascular adaptation as a function of the intensity and duration of training of young women. *Can J Appl Sport Sci,* 8(4), 260-265, 1983.

33. Marti, B., Abelin, T. and Minder, C.E. Relationship of training and life-style to 16-km running time of 4000 joggers. *Int J Sports Med,* 9, 85-91, 1988.

34. Milesis, C.A., Pollock, M.L., Bah, M.D., Ayres, J.J., Ward, A. and Linnerud, A.C. Effects of different duration's of physical training on cardiorespiratory function, body composition, and serum lipids. *Res Q,* 47, 716-725, 1976.

35. Mikesell, K.A., Dudley, G.A. Influence of intense endurance training on aerobic power of competitive distance runners. *Med Sci Sports Exerc,* 16(4), 371-375, 1984.

36. Moffatt, J.R., Stamford, B.A. and Neill, R.D. Placement of tri-weekly training sessions: importance regarding enhancement of aerobic capacity. *Res Q,* 48(3), 583-591, 1977.

37. Murphy, M.H. and Hardman, A.E. Training effects of short and long bouts of brisk walking in sedentary women. *Med Sci Sports Exerc,* 30(1), 152-157, 1998.

38. Murrey, T.D., Zingraf, S.A. and Shea, C. The relationship of selected training variables on performance in marathon running. *Med Sci Sports Exerc (Abstract),* 12, 81, 1980.

39. Nordesjö, L.O. The effect of quantified training of the capacity for short and prolonged work. *Acta Physiol Scand* 90, Suppl. 405, 1974.

40. Pollock, M.L., Cureton, T.K. and Greninger, L. Effects of frequency of training on working capacity, cardiovascular function, and body composition of adult men. *Med Sci Sports,* 1(2), 70-74, 1969.

41. Pollock, M.L., Miller, H.S., Linnerud, A.C. and Cooper, K.H. Frequency of training as a determinant for improvement in cardiovascular function and body composition of middle-aged men. *Arch Phys Med Rehabil,* 56, 141-145, 1975.

42. Rusko, H. The effect of training on aerobic power characteristics of young cross-country skiers. *J Sports Sci,* 5, 273-286, 1987.

43. Rusko, H., Rahkila, P. Effect of increased intensity of training on maximum oxygen uptake and muscular performance of young female cross-country skiers. *Med Sport,* 14, 187-194, 1981.

44. Saltin, B., Blomqvist, G., Mitchell, J.H., Johnson, R.L.Jr., Wildenthal, K. and Chapman, C.B. Response to exercise after bed rest and after training. *Circulation,* 38(5 Suppl.), VII, 1-78, 1968.

45. Schantz, P., Henriksson, J. and Jansson, E. Adaptation of human skeletal muscle to endurance training of long duration. *Clin Physiol* 3, 141-151, 1983.

46. Scrimgeour, A.G., Noakes, T.D., Adams, B. and Myburgh, K. The influence of weekly training distance on fractional utilization of maximum aerobic capacity in marathon and ultramarathon runners. *Eur J Appl Physiol,* 55, 202-209, 1986.

47. Sharkey, B.J. Intensity and duration of training and the development of cardiorespiratory endurance. *Med Sci Sports,* 2(4), 197-202, 1970.

48. Shephard, R. Intensity, duration and frequency of exercise as determinants of the response to a training regime. *Int Z angew Physiol einschl Arbeitsphysiol,* 26, 272-278, 1968.

49. Sjödin, B. and Jacobs, B. Onset of blood lactate accumulation and marathon running performance. *Int J Sports Medicine,* 2, 23-26, 1981.

50. Sjödin, B., Jacobs I. and Svedenhag, J. Changes in blood lactate accumulation (OBLA) and enzymes after training at OBLA. *Eur J Appl Physiol,* 49, 45-57, 1982.

51. Sjödin, B. and Svedenhag J. Applied Physiology of marathon running. *Sports Med,* 2, 83-99, 1985.

52. Slovic, P. Empirical study of training and performance in the marathon. *Res Q,* 48, 769-777, 1977.

53. Smith, D.J. and Wenger, H.A. The 10-day aerobic mini-cycle: The effects of interval or continuous training at two different intensities. *J Sports Med,* 21, 390-394, 1981.

54. Svedenhag, J. and Sjödin, B. Physiological characteristics of elite male runners in an off season. *Can J Appl Spt Sci,* 10(3), 127-133, 1985.
55. Tabata, I., Nishimura, K., Kauzaki, M., Hirai, Y., Ogita, F., Miyachi, M. and Yamamoto, K. Effects of moderate-intensity endurance and high-intensity intermittent training on anaerobic capacity and VO_2-max. *Med Sci Sports Exerc,* 28 (10), 1327-1330, 1996.
56. Weltman, A., Weltman, J.Y., Schurrer, R., Evans, W.S., Veldhuis, D. and Rogol, A.D. Endurance training amplifies the pulsatile release of growth hormone: effects of training intensity. *J Appl Physiol,* 72(6), 2188-2196, 1992.
57. Wenger, H.A. and Macnab, R.B.J. Endurance training: The effects of intensity, total work, duration and initial fitness. *J. Sports Med,* 15, 199-211, 1975.
58. Westgarth-Taylor, C., Hawley, J.A., Rickard, S., Myburgh, K.H., Noakes, T.D. and Dennis, S.C. Metabolic and performance adaptations to interval training in endurance-trained cyclists. *Eur J Appl Physiol,* 75, 298-304, 1997.
59. Weston, A.R., Myburgh, K.H., Lindsay, F.H., Dennis, S.C., Noakes, T.D. and Hawley, J.A. Skeletal muscle buffering capacity and endurance performance after high-intensity training by well-trained cyclists. *Eur J Appl Physiol,* 75, 7-13, 1997.
60. Yeager, S.A. and Brynteson, P. Effects of varying training periods on the development of cardiovascular efficiency of college women. *Res Q,* 41(4), 589-592, 1970.

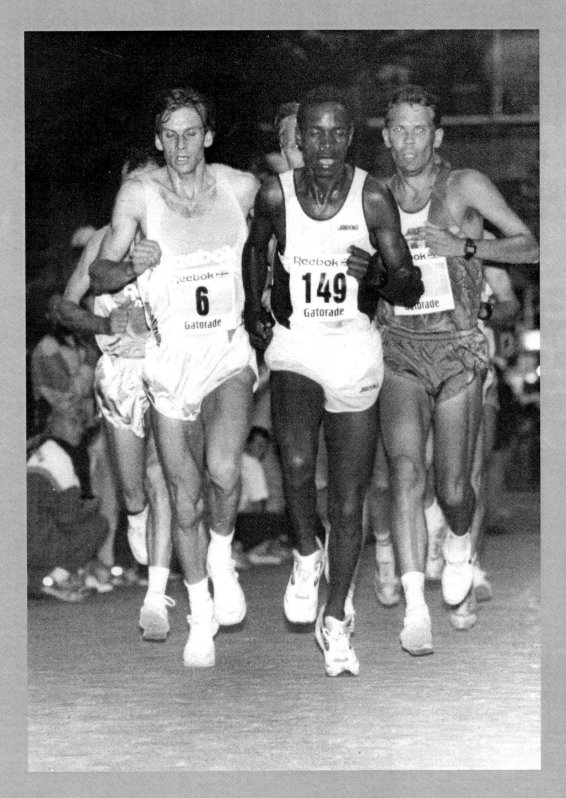

Training volume and intensity

Leif Inge Tjelta and Eystein Enoksen

Synopsis

A review of relevant literature, current research and experience of famous coaches and athletes show that: The most successful long distance runners through the last 30 years run between 140-250 km per week. 5000 m and 10000 m runners do work loads between 160-200 km, while marathon runners in certain weeks have training volume up to 250 km per week. The best female long distance runners run the same amount of kilometre per week as the international elite for men. Several world class long distance runners claim that training intensity is equally important as training volume. However, athletes are responding differently to training and only a few athletes have got the genetic dispositions to become world class runners.

Introduction

In this article we will venture to give a survey of characteristics in the development of some training theories, theories which are at the basis of successful long distance runners in this century. Thereupon we will define the terms training volume and training intensity. In the paragraph on training volume we will try to show the amount of training done by some successful runners.

In conjunction with the term training intensity we will discuss in which way certain coaches and physiologists subdivide training zones as well as the effect of training in the various zones.

Finally, we will concentrate on the training of three female long distance runners, namely Grete Waitz, Ingrid Kristiansen and Sonia O'Sullivan. We will try to compare training volume as well as training intensity for these outstanding runners.

Historical review of training theories

The theories which form the basis for the training of long distance runners have undergone some changes over the last 70 years. These theories have been influenced as well by the ideas of some acknowledged coaches as by physiological research.

Coaches who have been associated with good athletes tend to become trend-setters for other contemporary coaches and athletes. Consequently, a historical review of the main development in training theory can thus be exemplified by the following coach athlete relations:

- 1920s - 1930s: Lauri Pikhala - Paavo Nurmi (Finland). They developed a system which was a precursor of interval training (6).
- 1930s: Woldemar Gerschler - Rudolf Harbig (Germany). Gerschler introduced the term „interval training" (6).
- 1940s - 1950s: Gøsta Holmer - Gunder Hägg and Arne Anderson (Sweden). These legendary Swedes developed „fartlek" as a training method (6).
- 1950s: Miholov Igloi - Sandor Iharos, Laszlo Tabori and Sandor Rozsnyi (Hungary). The Hungarian based his ideas on Gerschler's principles on interval training, but he differed from Gerschler by also using a higher training intensity. Igloi held the idea that the runner should train twice a day (6).
- 1960's: Ernest Van Aaken - Harold Norpoth (West Germany) built their training principles on the idea that long steady running ought to be the basis of efficient long distance training (42).
- 1960s: Arthur Lydiard - Peter Snell (New Zealand). The New Zealander had the philosophy that 800 m runners as well as marathon runners must have a basic training period rooted on long distance

running. During this period they were to run 160 km per week. Thereupon followed a period of hill running (6-8 weeks) and a period of 10-12 weeks of track training leading up to that „year's run" (25).

Several coaches have also been influenced by physiologists and research. Woldemar Gerschler is an example of this in close cooperation with the physiologist Herbert Reindell (6). Norpoth's coach Van Aaken had a background as a researcher (6). The research done by the Italian physiologist Conconi, who determined the anaerobic threshold by non-invasive field tests (7), is one of many examples of how physiological research was used by coaches and athletes.

Some athletes had also developed their training theories based on their own experience, without any strong influence of coaches and physiologists. The four-time Olympic champion Emil Zatopek may serve as an example of this. Zatopek would run more kilometres per week than top runners had done before him (21). Zatokpek, on one occasion, when pursuing a theory that running whilst holding his breath would enhance his competitive performance, he was found unconscious at the side of the road. He had been trying to beat his own record for the number of telephone poles he could pass.

With a basis in the examples above we will use the term experts for coaches and physiologists who have introduced theories and training methods in long distance running. These theories may be founded on practical experience as well as research.

Let us now have a closer look at what kind of training some recognised experts have advocated for long distance runners over the last two decades. We have chosen the following: Martin, D.E. USA and Coe, P., England (26); Gambetta, V., USA (12); Pisuke, A. and Nurmekivi, A., The Soviet Union (34); Karikosk, O., The Soviet Union (21); Bernard, A., Canada (2); Nurmekivi, A., The Soviet Union (31); van Dam, B., West Germany (43); van den Eynde. Belgium (44) and Steffney, M., West Germany (39).

Martin and Coe (26) refer to the book: „Training Distance Runners" which was written by the American physiologist David E. Martin and the English trainer Peter N. Coe, the father and coach of Sebastian Coe. The other experts have stated their views on long distance running in various articles in international periodicals.

We shall also be referring to some other experts.

To be able to evaluate differing theories and views on long distance running we consider it important to clarify what we as well as the experts understand with the very central terms: training volume and training intensity.

Training volume

The term training volume may have two meanings in training theory (13):

A. *The totality of training effort or work done per time unit* (day, week, month, year) Based on the principles of mechanics this means that
work = efficiency x time or: work = intensity x time.

B. *The duration, the extent or the totality of* measured in for instance the number of kilometres or miles per time unit (day, week, month or year).

The meaning in B is the one most widely used in international literature on running. This is also the meaning used by the above mentioned experts and as a basis for what is here mentioned about training volume. When we use the term training volume we will take it in meaning B. Nevertheless, the connection between intensity and time is always important, and there is no doubt that the amount of work is greater when you run a certain distance (e.g. 10 km) at a speed of 16 km per hour instead of at a speed of 14 km per hour.

The Estonian Olav Karikosk (21), who is particularly preoccupied with the relation between training volume and achievements, has collected such data for many of the world's best long distance runners. One of the most striking traits in the development in long distance training these last 50 years has been the sheer volume in training. The one responsible for the first big increase in training volume was Emil Zatopek. When Zatopek improved Gunder Hägg's world record by one second, from 13:58.2 to 13:57.2 min:s, he annually ran three to four times as many kilometres as Hägg had done. When Zatopek set his last world record in the 10000 m (28:54.2 min:s) in 1954, his annual training volume was 8086 kilometres.

Zatopek's record was beaten by the double Olympic champion from Melbourne in 1956, Vladimir Kuts, who, compared to Zatopek, reduced the training volume considerably and increased training intensity.

Kuts would run 5000-6000 kilometres per year when he was at his best. Pyotor Bolotnikov had similar training volumes the year he set his two world records on 10000 m: 28:18.8 (5700 km/year) and 28:18.2 min:s (6000 km/year).

Ron Clarke, who pushed Kuts and Bolotnikov out of the result lists, states that he was preoccupied neither with counting kilometres nor with filling in log books for his training. Clarke estimates that he averaged 160 kilometres per week in 1963 when he set his first 10000 m world record (28.15.6 min:s). Later on, however, he reduced the training volume and increased the intensity. Clarke emphasises that intensity is more important than volume, and that the achievements are improved through intense training, not through steady speed over innumerable kilometres.

The Kenyan top class runner Henry Rono, who set records in 3000 (7:32.1 min:s), 5000 (13:08.4), 10000 (27:22.4) and 3000 m steeple-chase (8:05.4) in 1978, averaged 150-170 km/ week, which also goes for the Ethiopian Miruts Yifter (Olympic gold in the 5000 metre and the 10000 m in 1980). The Englishman David Moorcroft, who ran the 5000 m in 13:00.41 min:s (world record) in 1982, on the average covered 150-160 km per week during the years 1981 and 1982. The European champion of 1982, the German Thomas Wessinghage, ran 130-140 km with intensive training per week (the article by Karikosk does not express what he means by "intensive").

Karikosk maintains that the results of his survey suggest that top results have been achieved with varying training volumes, and that the runners with the highest training volume frequently have suffered injuries. The Finns Juha Vaatainen (European champion in the 5000 and the 10000 m in 1971) and Kaarlo Maaninka (bronze – in the 5000 and silver medallist 10000 m in 1980) could be cited as examples of this. These two runners respectively covered 10000 km and 12000 km per year the years they took their medals. Lasse Viren ran 7390 km per year when he won the Olympic gold medal in 1972. When he repeated the feat four years later his annual training volume was nearly the same (7300 km), but the intensity was higher.

The Soviet runner Valery Abramov is mentioned in connection with those who run fast but with a relatively low kilometer volume; in 1981 he did 13:11.99 min:s on the 5000 m with a yearly training volume of 5900 kilometers.

Four Norwegian male long distance runners, Knut Kvalheim, Per Halle, Knut Børø and Arne Kvalheim, were competing at an international level in the seventies. They would run between 160 and 190 km in weekly average for the preparation period (November – April) during the years they achieved their best results in the 3000, 5000 and 10000 m. During the competition period (May – the end of August) the average training distance was lowered to 142-158 km per week (15).

Noakes (30) has also studied the training volume of some of the all-time top long distance runners. He concludes that the best runs were done by athletes who covered between 150-200 km per week. He further maintains that the best marathon runners as Kohlemainen, Nurmi, Zatopek, Peters, Edelen, Clayton, Shorter, de Castella, Salazar, Jones and Lopes were excellent track or cross country runners before having success in marathons.

With a basis in his survey Karikosk (21) claims that an increase in training volume will not necessarily lead to better achievements. Noakes (30) holds the same opinion. There are also other sides to training that should be emphasised. Training intensity is one of them. Karikosk and Noakes do, however, not have adequate data on the training intensity of their runners to make comparisons, or for that sake, draw any conclusions. Klemm (22) maintains that the training volume of a 10000 m elite runner should be between 150-200 km per week. For a marathon runner of international standing it ought to be somewhat higher (200-250 kilometres per week).

Steffney (39) states that the training volume for a long distance runner must be increased according to the improvements made by the athlete. Steffney recommends that the athletes who have realistic hopes of running the 10000 m in 28 minutes should run 180 km per week during the preparation period (October - March). Athletes who aim to do it in approximately 30 minutes should run 140 km per week. Steffney substantiates his training theories by listing athletes who have been training according to the directions he is outlining.

The last two decades international long distance runners have been greatly dominated by African runners. The Kenyan runners on a senior level run between 160-200 km per week (9), and the training volume of Moroccan runners (38) is about the same level. Kenyan as well as Moroccan long distance runners are recognised by the quality of their aerobic training. Moroccan runners do five sessions each week with hill running, interval running or fartlek during the winter season. The remaining nine weekly running sessions are 50-60 minutes distance running (38). The Kenyans mostly do distance running during the winter season (November – February). The intensity of the distance runs are very often close to the anaerobic threshold (9). The anaerobic threshold is the highest level of exercise where the energy needs for the organism can be covered exclusively by aerobic metabolism (26).

All long distance runners mentioned by Karikosk (21) and Noakes (30) in connection with the discussion on efficient training volume are men. Then we may apply question if this training volume should also be recommended for the best female runners. The British middle and long distance coach Norman Brook (6) maintains that female runners who want to make it to the top in long distance running must train just as much as the best men. Any differences in training volume should be related to training and achievement, not to differences in sex. The Italian long distance coach Giampaolo Lenzi (23) who was the coach of Laura Fogli, the silver medallist in the marathon in the European Championship in Ahtens in 1982, holds the same opinion. The Olympic champion at the 10000 m in 1988, Olga Bondarenko, would run 160-180 km for two out of three weeks during her basic training period. The third week she would reduce the training volume to 100-110 km (5).

According to the Portuguese long distance coach Pompilio Ferreira (11) Rosa Mota who was European champion in marathon in 1982, would run an average of 150 km per week in 1981-1982.

It has been claimed that the Chinese female long distance runners who in 1992 set world records in the 3000, 5000 and 10000 m, would run a marathon distance daily (42195 m) during their basic training period (24). This would correspond to approximately 295 km per week, a training volume which is considerably higher than what is recommended by the above mentioned experts.

To Van Dam (43) there does not seem to be any fundamental difference in the training of men and women. He does however underline the fact that the increased production of the female sex hormone in the week preceding the menstruation may result in lower achievements in this period. Jansson (17) states that opinions differ as to whether the potential for achievement fluctuates during the various phases of the menstrual period. According to Jansson (17) some studies show no difference. Jurkowski (18) on the other hand showed that the achievements were better and the level of blood lactate was lower during the last part of the menstrual period than during the first part.

Several studies have shown that there is a correlation between the degree and the frequency of menstrual irregularities and the training volume measured in kilometres per week (30). In a study (10) it was discovered that 43% of female athletes who ran more than 128 km per week had irregular menstruation. Furthermore there was a parallel relationship between lacking menstruation and weekly training volume. There is, however, no indication of an absolute kilometre level above which training will lead to a loss of menstruation. Which again means that there is great individual variation in the adaptation to training volume (30). Consequently, the mechanisms which cause great training volumes to influence the regularity of menstruation seem to be a combination of several factors (30).

Tomten (41) who has been doing research on osteoporosis among female long distance runners, found that menstrual irregularities are common with young female runners who develop osteoporosis. She also discovered an overrepresentation of menstrual irregularities among the best runners.

Several studies conclude that there is no connection between training and menstrual status for female runners (27, 36, 37, 45).

Training intensity

There are two ways to express training intensity (13):

A: *As an absolute entity.* In endurance sports training intensity will thus be defined as meters per second, kilometres per hour or $\dot{V}O_2$ per minute

B: *As a relative entity.* The work done is expressed in a percentage of what the athlete could achieve at the maximum of his or her training condition. In endurance sports it is usual to express training intensity in a percentage of: $\dot{V}O_2$-max, maximum HR (heart rate) speed and HR at the anaerobic threshold or at competition speed.

For the further discussion we shall be using Figure 1 as a point of departure in order to have an adequate system of reference. Figure 1 shows examples of a scale of intensity, and also how some parameters and training methods vary when the intensity increases. Figure 1 describes training intensity as a relative entity.

Work load	Very low	Low	Medium	High	Very high	Max
Personal feeling	Slow	Talking	Do not push Moderate effort	Pushes a lot. Short breathing Hard effort	Pushes hard Very hard effort	Maximal effort
Work intensity (% of max HR)	60 65 70 75		80 85	90	95 100	
Heart rate	120 134 148			162 (AT)	176 190 (max)	
Work intensity (% of max HR – resting HR)	45 50 55 60 65		70 75 80 85		90 95 100	
Work intensity (% of max oxygen uptake)	45 50 55 60 65		70 75 80 85 90		95 100	
Stroke volume (Heart)	Increasing	Maximum	Maximum		Maximum	
Stroke power (Heart)	Gradually increasing	Increasing	Maximum			
Musclefiber in use	I	I	I + II A	I +II A + II B →		
Dominating energy Demand in musclefiber	Fat	Aerobic glycolysis				Anaerobic glycolysis
Training methods used in the different intensity zones	Restitution Slow distance running	Easy distance running	Moderate distance running Fartlek Intervall training (long)	Fast distance running Intervall training (short) Anaerobic treshold training	Aerobic capacity training VO2 max Race pace (5000m-1500m)	Anaerobic Capacity Training Tempo Training (short)
Blood lactate (mmol•l^{-1})	0.5-1	1-1.5	1.5-2	2-4	4-8	8-20

Figure 1. An example of a scale of intensity for endurance training for a well trained athlete with a maximum heart frequency of 190 beats • min^{-1} and a rest frequency of 50 beats • min^{-1}. The figure generally illustrates how certain physiological parameters and training methods vary when intensity increases (13).

Most experts mentioned above divide long distance training into three zones of intensity, namely:

- *Aerobic intensity zone,* which corresponds to what we in Figure 1 have classified as very low, low and moderate work load. Exertions with moderate work load (70-80% of $\dot{V}O_2$-max) are however classified as aerobic/anaerobic training by experts like Pisuke and Nurmekivi (35).
- *Aerobic/anaerobic intensity zone,* which corresponds to high or very high work load (Figure 1).
- *Anaerobic intensity zone,* which corresponds to an area of intensity which in Figure 1 is classified as maximal work intensity. Some experts also place work intensities which in Figure 1 appear as very high, under the label anaerobic (33, 44).

Martin and Coe (26) divide efficient training into four zones of intensity. They also use different terms for these zones than the other authors. We will return to this later on.

Aerobic intensity zone

In this intensity zone the strain is 50-70/80% of the strain at $\dot{V}O_2$-max. This corresponds to figure 1 where low work load is defined as 50/55-65/70% of the strain at $\dot{V}O_2$-max, and that moderate work intensity is 65/70-80 of $\dot{V}O_2$-max. The concentration of blood lactate is below the anaerobic threshold (AT). With a reference to Figure 1 we see that the blood lactate concentration is estimated to be 1-2 mmol•l^{-1} at these levels of strain. Several experts quote higher values of lactate in this intensity zone. This can be ascribed to the fact that different testing procedures give different values of lactate (14).

Most training for long distance runners should be done in this zone of intensity according to the above mentioned experts. The length of the training sessions in the aerobic intensity zone are usually between 8 and 35 km. The training is most often in the form of continuous work over long distances. Training in this zone is frequently referred to as „basic training" or „conversational training" because it is steady enough to allow conversation while running. If the heart rate (HR) is taken as a measure of training intensity the heart rate is around 70-80% of maximum heart rate. This training will, according to Martin and Coe (26) have the following effects:

- It will serve to improve oxidative metabolic capabilities in cardiac muscle and those skeletal muscle cells that are activated (type 1 fibres).
- It provides a stimulus for improving joint and tendon strength without excessive impact stress, which would be the result at faster paces.
- Increases occur in the quantity of stored fuels (carbohydrates and fatty acids).
- It will lead to increase as well in number as in size of mitochondria in the stimulated muscle cells.
- Increasing blood volume and capillary density in trained muscle will improve O_2 delivery and CO_2 removal.
- The sustained increased venous return to the heart, particularly during longer runs, provides an initial stimulus toward enlarging ventricular chambers, eventually increasing stroke volume and permitting a given volume to be pumped at lower heart rate. This will lead to lower resting heart rate.

Martin and Coe maintain that running at a speed slower than 55% of the speed at $\dot{V}O_2$-max has little aerobic value. Pisuke and Nurmekivi (34) term training below 50% of $\dot{V}O_2$-max speeds as restitution training. Figure 1 defines training where the intensity is below 55% at the effort at $\dot{V}O_2$-max as restitution or training at very low intensity.

Aerobic / anaerobic intensity zone

Training in this intensity zone produces increased stimulation of heart and the cardiovascular system (26) Training in the aerobic / anaerobic intensity zone is also important as concerns the effect of training of those muscle cells that are above the strain level in the aerobic intensity zone (26). Running intensity in this zone covers speeds from somewhat lower to somewhat faster than the running speeds for the anaerobic threshold. (2, 26, 31, 34, 39, 43).

By applying the measuring method which is usually used in Norway today in order to determine the anaerobic threshold (AT), it was discovered that the eight best female long distance runners in Norway in 1994-1995 had an oxygen uptake at AT which was from 83-89% of $\dot{V}O_2$-max (40). The test is organised as a progressive running proceedure over five steps, where lactate, oxygen uptake and heart rate are measured at the end of each working load. Lactate measured at loads lower than AT are stable after 2-5 minutes. 5 minutes are chosen as working time. The first load is approximately 60% of the $\dot{V}O_2$-max load. For each increase in work load the oxygen uptake will be 6-7% higher and the heart frequency will increase with approximately ten beats per minute. The test contains of five different working loads. AT is set to be the running speed (km per hour), oxygen uptake and heart frequency which correlates to a lactate concentration in blood which is 1.5 mmol•l⁻¹ above the lovest measured test value (1). Bompa (4), Martin and Coe (26) and Nurmekivi (32) also claim that AT lies in this percentage area of $\dot{V}O_2$-max.

In Figure 1 we also see that the lactate value at AT is approximately 2.5 mmol•l⁻¹. Frequent measurements of the best female long distance runners in Norway during 1994-95 showed that their AT, measured by the measurement methods used in Norway today (1), lay about 2.05 and 2.72 mmol•l⁻¹ (40). Measurements for male runners generally show similar values. Some literature refers to other methods of measurements, which by using the same percentage of exertion, would have given an AT about 4 mmol•l⁻¹ (12, 26).

Martin and Coe (26) characterise training in the zone around AT as: anaerobic conditioning because training at speeds above the anaerobic threshold will result in a rapid concentration of lactate in the blood.

While Pisuke and Nurmekivi (34) say that speeds between 70-100% of $\dot{V}O_2$-max lie in this zone, this covers two of the zones in Coe and Martin's (26) system. In figure 1 this spans the three intensity zones; moderate, high and very high workload. All experts agree that training in the intensity zone 70-100% of the speed at $\dot{V}O_2$-max should contain continuous work as well as interval training.

Continuous work is an efficient form of training which corresponds to 70/75-85/90% of the speed at $\dot{V}O_2$-max. Other experts recommend both continuous work and long interval training in this intensity zone. (2, 13, 34, 39).

There is general agreement that interval training is an efficient form of training when the intensity of the training is between 90-100% of the speed at $\dot{V}O_2$-max. According to Martin and Coe (26) these are speeds that correspond to the speed of the distances 1000-3000 m. They call training in this training zone aerobic capacity training and recommend long interval training (distances from 800-3000 m). The total running distances should be from 6-8 km. This corresponds well with Bernard (2) who says that 8-9 x 800 m with 2-3 minute recovery is what he recommends for training at 10000 speed. Steffney (39) also recommends forms of training at a level of intensity which corresponds to this.

Coe and Martin (26) list the following training effects in the intensity zone close to the anaerobic threshold corresponding to 75-90% of the speed at $\dot{V}O_2$-max:
• It will develop stamina.
• ST fibres and some FT fibres (Type IIa) will be developed.
• Increased heart chamber size.
• Increased stroke volume.
• Increased oxidative/glycolytic enzymes.
• Increased blood volume.

Nurmekivi (31) states that continuous running at steady state pace in the area close to the athlete's anaerobic threshold has the following effects:
• The improvement of blood supply through the development of capillaries.
• An increase in the number of capillaries.
• The capacity to eliminate accumulated lactate faster during work.
• An increase in the contraction capacity of the heart muscle.

If the effect of the training is in the area from 90-100% of the speed at $\dot{V}O_2$-max Martin and Coe (26) claim that the physiological adaptations resulting from this kind of training include:
• Increased glycolytic enzymes in working muscles.
• Some increase in blood buffering ability.
• Some increase in neurological recruitment.
• ST and FT fibre development.
• Development of speed.

Anaerobic intensity zone

Training with an intensity of 100% or more of the speed at $\dot{V}O_2$-max is defined as anaerobic training by all experts. In Figure 1 this is classified as training which gives the highest strain in this area; very high work intensity as well as maximum work intensity. There is, however, some disagreement concerning the extent as well as the actual exaction of such training for long distance runners.

Gambetta (12) calls anaerobic training „repetition training". This is not to be confused with interval training. The training distances should be about ½ to ¾ of the competition distances. Between the repetitions there should be long breaks and good restitution. Van den Eynde (44) on the other hand recommends high intensity and short breaks to develop anaerobic endurance. As examples of such training he mentions:

- Speed running from 200-1000 m with short breaks (100-200 m jogging)
- Variations in speed (ins and outs) for 1000-2000 m in one or two series with 4-6 minute serial pauses.
- Several repetitions with hill running from 200-800 m, where running down the hill again to the starting point constitutes the pause.
- Speed training after a spell of aerobic training, or separate speed training. 80-150 m sprint with short pauses between are those recommended.

Pisuke (33) holds the opinion that anaerobic training should constitute about 5-10% of the annual total training volume of a senior athlete. But then Pisuke also considers training intensities from 95-100% of $\dot{V}O_2$-max as anaerobic training. Junior runners should hold a lower percentage. Together with Gambetta he also recommends repetitions. In addition he believes that interval training, hill running, and several variations of jumps are potentially efficient forms of training.

Bernard (2) also underlines that training in speeds which are 10-15% higher than competitive speeds must be included in the training. Bernard quotes no specific percentage of training as a recommended level of intensity.

Nurmekivi (31) claims that anaerobic training must be related to whether the runner has speed (has a large percentage of fast muscle fibres (FT)) or endurance (a majority of slow muscle fibres (ST)). Endurance runners can use longer distances in interval as well as repetition training, but they should be careful about intensive interval training. Nurmekivi (31) recommends one to three track sessions per week. We should also be aware that training repetition on grass or trail is less psychologically stressing than track training.

van Dam (43) maintains the importance of training one weekly session with high intensity all through the winter. In this way you avoid having to do a great number of intensive 200 and 300 meters just before the track season.

Steffney (39) believes that particularly 10000 m runners should be careful about intensive track training during the season of competitions. The danger lies in the emphasis on developing speed to the detriment of endurance. Steffney suggests speed alternations (20 x 50 m) as well as sessions at competitive speed for 1500, 3000, 5000 and 10000 m as forms of anaerobic training.

Martin and Coe (26) say that the purpose of anaerobic capacity training is to improve speed and strength. Furthermore such training improves the ability to take speed changes and the ability to finish a race well. The 1500 m as well as the 3000 m are run with over 100% of the speed at $\dot{V}O_2$-max, and consequently it is important to develop the ability to perform with a steadily growing level of blood lactate in the muscles that are being strained. Martin and Coe (26) also maintain that the distances 5000 and 10000 m will be run most successfully by the runners who in addition to maintaining a high speed and a low production of blood lactate at the final stages of the run, can add an anaerobic element the last stretch before the finish.

Training sessions which are intended to increase the anaerobic capacity must be executed at great speed over relatively short distances. Coe and Martin (26) recommend running distances of 200-800 m and a total training volume per session of 2400-4000 m.

Case studies

At the end of this article we will analyse the training done by Grete Waitz and Ingrid Kristiansen when they were the best long distance runners in the world. Furthermore we will discuss the training of Sonia O'Sullivan who was the best long distance runner in 1995 and the world champion on the 5000 m. She had a set-back in 1997 and then she managed to get a formidable comeback as the double world champion in cross country as well as winner of 5000 m and 10000 m in the European championship in 1998. We will try to evaluate the training of each runner individually during one of the seasons she was at the top. As for Ingrid and Grete we will try to comment on their training the years leading up to the year we have chosen to concentrate on. We will also compare the training of these runners, as well as compare it to the long distance training which is recommended by today's experts.

Our information concerning Grete Waitz' training is from her training log from 1973/74, from telephone conversations with her and from the previous Norwegian national coach Kai Møller (28, 29). With a basis in Grete's training logs he has established a system of the training that Grete did when she was a track runner. We have gained much of our knowledge concerning Grete's training prior to being a senior during conversations with Grete.

Johan Kaggestad has let us study Ingrid Kristiansen's log book from 1985/86. When he was a national coach he systematised Ingrid's training between 18 November 1985 and 26 October 1986 (19, 20). Further information about Ingrid's training in the years preceding the 1986 season have been gained during conversations with her.

Sonia O'Sullivan was Grete Waitz' neighbour and friend in Gainesville, USA. The information we have on Sonia O'Sullivan has been relayed to us by Grete Waitz.

Grete Waitz

Grete Waitz started athletics at the age of 12. She would compete in sprint, jumping and throwing events up till the age of 14. At the age of 15 she for the first time took part in races over 200 m. She ran her first 800 m at the age of 16. At this age she would train 5 times a week. She did interval training and steady long runs up to 8-10 km. Grete says she trained a lot with the boys and that training intensity was relatively high already at the age of 17-19. „I was able to do a kilometre in four minutes sharp at an age of 18-19 years without making much of an effort." As a 19 year old girl Grete held the following personal records: 800 m 2:05.7 min:s, 1500 m 4:17.0 min:s, and 1.61 m in high jump.

„I believe the reason why I was able to take a lot of tough training as an adult without the support of a medical team was that I had established a sound basis through all-round training during my youth".

Training volume and training intensity as a senior athlete
From the autumn of 1973 Grete's training changed. The total volume was increased. The percentage of her intensive sessions was very much

lowered, and sprint training was dropped. Two-three times a week she would run twice a day, thus contributing to the increase in the total number of kilometres (28). Kai Møller (28) says that the training in 1973/74 represents the shift to long distance training. Her training prior to 73/74 is characterised as 800 m training (28). Eight of September 1974 Grete was number three in the 1500 m in the European championship. There is a comparison of Grete's training frequency (number of sessions) in 1971/72 and 1973/74 in Table 1, and the various types of training for the years 1971/72 and 1973/74 are shown in Table 2. Møller comments: „In the season 1971/72 Grete did mainly intensive training all through the year. The training is particularly intensive during the season of competitions. A great number of competitions are not included in the table.

Table 1. Grete Waitz' training frequency during the seasons 1971/72 and 1973/74.

Selected months	November	February	April	July	August
No. of sessions 1971/72:	28	32	30	21	31
No. of sessions 1973/74:	40	38	36	41	42

Data from 28.

In 1973/74 all the year is dominated by long steady training Table 2. Note in particular the month of September with important competitions, where as much as 78% is long runs. Both July and August have 68% long runs".

By surveying Grete's training diary for 1973/74 we find that her weekly training volume is between 80 and 116 km. The volume is somewhat higher during the summer season than in the winter. This is due to the fact that she during May-September more frequently runs twice a day than what she did during the period November 1973 till April 1974. The volume was reduced to 58.5 km the week before the European Championship.

During 27 consecutive weeks from 1 January 1974 she runs an average of 90 km per week. During the same time span in 1973 she would run 73.8 km per week.

Grete's training diaries reveal that 1974 was the year she hit upon her particular form of training. The ensuing years she increased the

Table 2. Types of training during the seasons 1971/72 and 1973/74 in percentage of total training.

Selected months

Types of training	November		February		April		July		August		September	
	1971	1973	1972	1974	1972	1974	1972	1974	1972	1974	1972	1974
long run over 10km.	28%	60%	28%	63%	23%	25%	9%	24%	16%	38%	----	43%
long run below 10km.	14%	15%	15%	18%	3%	25%	19%	39%	0%	30%	----	35%
fartlek	18%	5%	8%	3%	24%	9%	9%	5%	6%	0%	----	0%
long interval	3%	5%	18%	6%	10%	9%	5%	5%	0%	0%	----	0%
short interval	21%	7.5%	18%	10%	13%	19%	14%	11%	13%	11%	----	0%
anaerobic	0%	0%	0%	0%	0%	0%	12%	4%	35%	11%	----	0%
hill running	0%	0%	0%	0%	10%	3%	0%	0%	0%	0%	----	0%
competitions	0%	0%	3%	0%	7%	6%	24%	10%	19%	12%	----	11%
skiing	0%	0%	0%	0%	0%	6%	0%	0%	0%	0%	----	0%
strength	14%	7.5%	5%	0%	10%	0%	0%	0%	0%	0%	----	0%
sprint	0%	0%	5%	0%	0%	0%	8%	0%	6%	0%	----	0%

Data from 28.

training gradually. In 1975 her average training volume for the 25 weeks after 1 January was 132 km per week. This season Grete achieved: 3000 m in 8:46.6 min:s and the 1500 m in 4:07.5 min:s. From 1 January 1976 she averaged 160 km per week during the first 25 weeks of the year (29).

This was to remain her training volume until 1978/79, the year she had her best track runs; 4:00.6 min:s at the 1500 m in 1978 and 8:31.75 min:s at the 3000 m in 1979. She maintains that her speed during the long runs was relatively high. Grete's training diaries do, however, not contain any information about kilometre speed nor heart frequency during the long runs.

Grete tells that during the years as a marathon runner she did not have any noticeable increase in the training volume. Some of the long runs would however be very long and calm. This is confirmed by Kai Møller (28). Her training rhythm is exemplified by the following sessions from her diary for 1974 shown in Table 3.

Table 3. Different training weeks for Grete Waitz in 1974.

One training week in February 1974

Monday	4 February	Long run	14 km
Tuesday	5 February	Long run	14 km
Wednesday	6 February	Long run/with speed inkrease	14 km
Thursday	7 February	Long run	14 km
Friday	8 February	a) 4 x 1000 m, recovery 1 min	
		b) Long run	6 km
Saturday	9 February	Intervals 25 x 300 m, recovery 15 s	
Sunday	10 February	a) Long run	10 km
		b) Long run	10 km

One week of training in August 1974

Thursday	1 August	a) Long run 30 min	
		b) Fartlek	12 km
Friday	2 August	a) Long run	6 km
		b) Long run (last 5 km fast)	11 km
Saturday	3 August	a) Long run	7 km
		b) Short intervals 2 x 15 x 200 m, recovery 10-15 s.	
Sunday	4 August	a) Long run	7 km
		b) Long run	12 km
Monday	5 August	Tempo/distance at track: 1000 m (2:50), 600 m (1:37), 300 m (43.2) recovery 7:30 min.	
Tuesday	6 August	Long run	14 km
Wednesday	7 August	Short interval 2 x 12 x 150 m, recovery 10-15 s. Serial pause 5 min	

The last 2 weeks before the European Championship in Rome 1974

Friday	23 August	a) Long run	7 km
		b) Long run	13 km
Saturday	24 August	a) Long run	7 km
		b) Long run	13 km

Sunday	25 August	a) Long run	7 km
		b) Long run	13 km
Monday	26 August	a) Track:	
		1000 m (2:47.5 min:s) 600 m (1:36.1 min:s),	
		300 m 43.6 s), recovery 7:30 min.	
Tuesday	27 August	a) Long run	7 km
		b) Long run	13 km
Wednesday	28 August	No training due to infection of right leg	
Thursday	29 August	Jogging for 20 min	
Friday	30 August	Long run	13 km
Saturday	31 August	Track: 1000 m (2:42.6 min:s)	
		600 m (1:34.9 min:s) 300 m (43.1 s)	
		recovery 7.30 min.	
Sunday	1 Septmber	Long run	8 km
Monday	2 Septmber	Fartlek	11 km
Tuesday	3 Septmber	Long run	8 km
Wednesday	4 Septmber	Short interval: 12 x 150 m + 10 x	
		100 m, recovery 10-15 s. Serial	
		pause 5 min.	
Thursday	5 Septmber	25 min jogging + couple of hills	
Friday	6 Septmber	a) 4-5 km jogging	
		b) European Championship 1500 m	
		heat 4:11.5 min:s	
Saturday	7 Septmber	25 min jogging + couple of extra turns	
Sunday	8 Septmber	European Championship 1500 m final,	
		number 3. 4:05.2 min:s	
Monday	9 Septmber	Long run	8 km

Ingrid Kristiansen

Ingrid who was born in 1956 tells that she already in pre-school age would run and go for long walks in the fields, on foot as well as on skis. She continued doing this until she was 15/16 yr. She says that when she at an age of 15 yr took part in the first athletics training she experienced interval training emphasising time as very stressing. As a 15 yr old she did the 1500 m in 4:22.0 min:s. Her basis was varied aerobic training. Ingrid took part in competitions for a long time, at a high level, both in cross country skiing and in running. She won several national championships in skiing relay. She was also a member of the national team.

The season 1986

In 1985 Ingrid set the world record at the London Marathon with the time: 2:21:06 h:min:s. Her training for the 1986 season was aimed at the 10000 m in the European Championship in Germany 30th August. During the 1986 season Ingrid set world records both in the 5000 m (14:37.33 min:s) and the 10000 m (30:13.76 min:s). She became the European champion in the 10000 m and set personal records in the 1500 m as well as the 3000 m. During the 1986 season she took part in 28 competitions including two marathons.

Training volume

During the 49 weeks from 18th November 1985 until 26th October 1986 Ingrid had a total training volume of 7625 km (20). This amounts to 155 km per week.

Of the total annual training volume of 7625 kilometres, 565 kilometre was skiing (7.4%) and 114 km (1.5%) was cycling. Figure 2 shows the training volume per week in this period.

Training intensity

Aerobic training

6701 km (87.9%) of Ingrid's total training volume of 7625 km was aerobic training. From her training diaries we understand that this was mainly training in the area 55-75% of the speed at $\dot{V}O_2$-max.

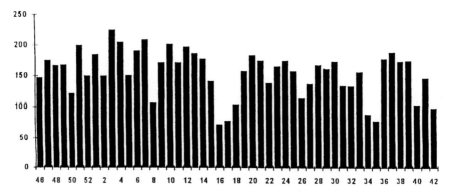

Figure 2. Training volume, measured in km • week^{-1}, during different weeks from 18 November, 1985 until 26 October 1986 for Ingrid Kristiansen. Data from 20.

Aerobic/anaerobic training

357 km (4.7%) was run in 39 sessions with a speed between 3:10 and 3:40 min:s per km. These sessions were executed with continuous work over distances of 3-23 km. Johan Kaggestad classifies this training as anaerobic threshold training. This corresponds well with the terminology used by Martin and Coe (26). Our interpretation of Martin and Coe gives us reason to classify this training as 70-85/90% of the speed at $\dot{V}O_2$-max. Figure 1 classifies this training as moderate and high work intensity. Most coaches and physiologist would classify this as aerobic/anaerobic training.

265 km(3.5%) in 45 sessions are classified as aerobic quality training by Kaggestad (aerobic capacity training; 26). This training was executed as various forms of interval training. It can be classified as in the upper part of aerobic/anaerobic zone of intensity. The speed was 85/90-100% at the speed of $\dot{V}O_2$-max. According to Figure 1 this is training with high and very high work intensity. These are speeds which correspond to the competition speed of the distances from 3000 m to ½ marathon (26) The total training in the aerobic/anaerobic intensity zone is then 622 km (8.2%).

Anaerobic training

Only a relatively low part, 28.3 km (0.37%) in 10 running sessions, was executed as anaerobic training, i.e. training where the speed is higher than the speed at $\dot{V}O_2$-max. In addition Ingrid would be running sprint strides of 60-100 m at high speed after having ended her other forms of training. She ran 166 sessions with a total of 1162 strides. This constitutes 9.3 km (0.12%). These 9.3 km with strides are classified as alactic anaerobic training (16).

Competitions

Ingrid took part in 28 competitions. The length varied from 1500 m to marathon. The total length of the competitions was 273.8 km which constitute 3.6% of her total kilometre volume.

Strength training

Between 18 November 1985 and 9 June 1986 Ingrid executed 37 sessions of strength training. These were sessions from 10 to 15 minutes with general strength training to one weekly session with aerobics lasting 70-80 min.

Training suppleness
During the period 18 November 1985 and 3 August 1986 Ingrid did 65 sessions of training, variations of jumps. They lasted from 10 to 15 min.

Hill running
Ingrid did 5 sessions of hill running over the mentioned 49 weeks. These sessions have already been included under the heading aerobic/anaerobic training.

Sonia O'Sullivan

Sonia O'Sullivan became the 1995 world champion on the 5000 m and she won the world cup. As previously mentioned she won the short as well as the long cross country distances in the world championship in 1998, she also won 5000 m and 10.000 m in the European championship this year. The training data presented in Table 4 are three representative weeks of 1994/95.

Table 4. Training of Sonia O'Sullivan 1994-1995.

End of November (London Base, Teddington)

Sunday	long steady run 1 hour 45 min, appr. 15-16 miles	
Monday	Session 1	10 miles steady
	Session 2	5 miles steady + circular training
Tuesday	Session 1	10 x hill runs (appr. 1 min duration)
	Session 2	7 miles + weights
Wednesday	Session 1	10 miles steady
	Session 2	5 miles steady
Thursday	Session 1	6 miles steady
	Session 2	Cricket field session. (1/2 mile + 1 mile) x 2 with 1 min recovery
Friday	Session 1	11 miles steady
	Session 2	5 miles steady
Saturday	Session 1	7 miles fast, time 39:12 min:s (3:32 min•km^{-1}) run in a park.

Total weekly volume: 100 miles

February/March (Australia)

Sunday		Long steady run 1 hour 50 min, 15-16 miles
Monday	Session 1	10 miles
	Session 2	5-6 miles + weights
Tuesday	Session 1	3 miles steady
	Session 2	track session: 5 x 1000 m. Time 2:50 min:s. Recovery: 120 s.
	Session 3	5-6 miles steady
Wednesday	Session 1	9 miles steady
	Session 2	5-6 miles steady
Thursday	Session 1	Hill runs. 10 x 65 s.
	Session 2	6 miles steady
Friday	Session 1	9 miles steady
	Session 2	5-6 miles steady + weight training
Saturday	Session 1	3 miles steady
	Session 2	Track session. 3 x (4x400 m). Time 62-65 s. Recovery: 1 min
	Session 3	5 miles steady

July /August (Teddington London)

Sunday	Session 1	From 45 to 60 min steady runs
Monday	Session 1	6 miles steady
	Session 2	6 miles steady
Tuesday	Session 1	15 to 20 min steady runs
	Session 2	Track session. 1200 m (3:15 min:s) 1000 m (2:45), 800 m (2:08), 600 m (1:35), 400 m (1:00), 200 m (0:28) (recovery are not quoted)
	Session 3	4 miles steady
Wednesday	Session 1	6 miles steady
	Session 2	5-6 miles
Thursday	Session 1	15 to 20 min steady run
	Session 2	Track session. 2 x (4x300 m). Time 46-47 s. Recovery: 1 min
	Session 3	4 miles steady
Friday	Session 1	20 min steady
	Session 2	20-30 min jogging + some hill runs
Saturday	Session 1	3-4 miles steady
	Session 2	Competition (1500, 3000 or 5000 m).

Training volume
During the period November until the beginning of May O'Sullivan would usually run 100 miles (160 km) per week. The highest distance that Sonia O'Sullivan covered during one week of 1995 was 112 miles (180 km). During the competition period she ran 72-75 miles (115-120 km) per week.

Training intensity
According to Grete Waitz (1995) O'Sullivan does her steady long runs with a speed of about 3:45 and 3:50 min•km^{-1}. To O'Sullivan these would constitute training in the boarder area between low and moderate work intensity (Figure 1). The longest trips on Sundays during basic training periods are calmer; 4:00-4:10 min•km^{-1}. This is training with low work intensity (Figure 1).

Winter training 1994-1995
The Saturday sessions that O'Sullivan does in her winter training are with high work intensity.
Session 1 Tuesday (10 x hill runs) and session 2 Thursday ((½ miles +1 mile) x 2) we would estimate to be training in the boarder area between high and very high work intensity (Figure 1).

Training during the spring of 1995
Two weekly sessions during the period February/March were executed with very high work intensity. These sessions are the session 2 on Tuesday (5x1000 m, Time: 2:50 min:s) and the session 2 on Saturday (track session 3 x (4x400 m), time: 62-65 min:s). Session 1 on Thursday (Hill session 10 x 65 s) is training in the boarder area between high and very high work intensity (Figure1).

Summer training 1995
In addition to one weekly competition during the summer of 1995 O'Sullivan trained two sessions per week with very high work intensity. These were done on the track Tuesday and Wednesday in July/August.

Similarities and differences in the training of Grete Waitz, Ingrid Kristiansen and Sonia O'Sullivan

Training volume

We find the highest weekly training volumes with Ingrid Kristiansen who competed in the longest distances. During the one week 13th - 19th January 1986 she had a total training volume of 225 km. It should be mentioned that 80 of these 225 km were performed on skis. In addition to the fact that Ingrid did great parts of her aerobic winter training on skis she would also do much training on the treadmill; over a period of 49 weeks she did 110 training sessions on the treadmill.

Sonia O'Sullivan (1995) and Grete Waitz (1976) had 180 km as their highest weekly training volumes. There is little difference in the average weekly training volume of these three athletes: Ingrid held an average of 155 km (average for 49 weeks), Grete had 160 km (average for 25 weeks) and Sonia O'Sullivan did 140-150 km per week. When you compare the training volume of these three female runners with that of the best male long distance runners, it corresponds to the volume that Karikosk (21), Noakes (30) and Klemm (22) maintain is the efficient level. Ingrid's total annual volume, 7625 km, is very close to that of Lasse Virén who in 1972 and 1976 covered 7390 km and 7300 km. In other words, there do not seem to be any substantial differences in the training volumes of men and women at the top international level.

Training intensity

When you compare the training of Grete Waitz (1976), Ingrid Kristiansen (1986) and Sonia O'Sullivan (1995) several similarities are apparent:

They all did 2 daily sessions and they all had 2-3 weekly training sessions in the aerobic/anaerobic zone of intensity. Further, their aerobic training, which constituted 80-90% of their total training, was of a high quality. Ingrid's training, however, contained less track training than that of the other two. They all three did strength training, but Sonia was the only one to use weights.

The distribution of training in the various zones of intensity corresponds well with what is recommended by van den Eynde (44), Steffney (39), Nurmekivi (31) and Pisuke (33).

With Grete and Ingrid we find similarities in training influences during their adolescence. They both did an extensive range of sports. Grete did sprint, jumping and throwing, and she played handball during her early youth. Ingrid trained skiing and running. There is one difference between the two in the fact that up till senior level Grete did more anaerobic training than Ingrid. The latter got her basic training through aerobics, ski training and runs in the forests. Grete achieved her best times on the 1500 m and the 3000 m. She was also best on the 400 m and the 800 m. Ingrid was the best on the longest distances. These are differences which may be ascribed to the differences in training during their teens and/or „genetic differences". It is however important to underline the fact that both Ingrid and Grete did 150-160 km in weekly average during the years they were doing their best 1500 and 3000 m runs.

References

1. Bahr, R., Hallen, J. & Medbø, J.I. *Testing av idrettsutøvere.* Oslo: Universitetsforlaget 1991.
2. Bernard, A.: Training for Aerobic Fitness. *Track and Field Journal,* 20, April, 1983.
3. Bouchard, C., Boulay, M.R., Simoneau, J.A., Lortie, G. & Perusse, L.: Heredity and trainability of aerobic and anaerobic performances. An update. *Sports Med.* 5: 69-73, 1986.
4. Bompa, T.O.: Physiological intensity values employed to plan endurance training. New Studies in Athletics, Vol. 4, No. 1., 1989.
5. Bondarenko, V.: How to win olympic gold medal in women's 10000 m. *XVIth E.A.C.A. Congress.* Endurance running 17.-21.01.1991. Finnish Sports Institute, Vierumaki, Finland, 1991.
6. Brook, N.: *Endurance Running Events.* British Athletic Federation, 1992.
7. Conconi, F., Ferrari, M., Ziglio, P. G., Drogetti, P. and Codeca, L.: Determination of the anaerobic threshold by non-invasive field test in runners. *J. Appl. Physiol.* vol.52, no 4: 869-873, 1982.
8. Evertsen, F.: Kilometersankerne, en saga blott? *Kondis* nr.3, mai/juni. 1995.
9. Evertsen, F.: Kenyansk langdistansetrening. *Idrettsmagasinet* nr.1, august 1998.
10. Feicht, C. B., Johnson, T. S., Martin, B. J., Sparkes, K. E. and Wagner, W. W.: Secondary amenorrhoea in athletes. *Lancet.* 2: 1145-1146, 1978.
11. Ferreira, P.: Experience in Oporto. *XII European Coaches Association.* Acoteias Portugal, 22.01-25.01, 1983.
12. Gambetta, V.: Distance Running Training. *Track and Field Quarterly Rev.,* Vol.79, No.3., 1979.
13. Gjerset, A. (red.): *Idrettens Treningslære.* Universitetsforlaget, Oslo, 1992.
14. Gjerset, A.; Johansen, E. og Moser T.: Aerobe og anaerobe arbeidskrav i kortidsorientering. *Idrettsmagasinet* nr. 1. august, 1998.

15. Husby, S. R.: En analyse av treningsarbeidet til fire norske langdistanseløpere: Knut Kvalheim, Per Halle, Knut Børø og Arne Kvalheim. *Fordypningsoppgave (Friidrett) våren 1982. 1. årig mellomfagstillegg i idrett.* Norges Idrettshøgskole, 1982.

16. Janssen, P. G. J. M.: *Trening, melkesyre, hjertefrekvens.* Universitetsforlaget, Oslo, 1993.

17. Jansson, E.: Kvinnor och aerob arbeidsførmåga. *Konditionsträning.* Red.: Forsberg, A. og Saltin, B. Idrottens Forskningsråd / Sveriges Riksidrottsførbund, 1988.

18. Jurkowski et al.: *Can. Journal of Applied Sports Science.* 7: 85-88, 1982.

19. Kaggestad, J.: So trainiert Ingrid Kristiansen 1986. *Leichtathletik.* 38: 831-834, 1987a.

20. Kaggestad, J.: En systematisering av treninga til Ingrid Kristiansen i sesongen 1986. *Upublisert materiale,* 1987b.

21. Karikosk, O.: Training Volume in Distance Running. *Modern Athlete and Coach.* Vol.23, No.2, April, 1985.

22. Klemm, W.: Energy Supply Differences in 10000 m and Marathon Runs. *Long Distances.* Edited by Jarver, J. Tafnews Press, 1989.

23. Lenzi, G.: The Womens Marathon: Preparing for an important event in the season. *XII Congress European Coaches Association.* Acoteias Portugal. 22/1-25/1, 1983.

24. Lier, A.: Trening av toppidrettsutøvere i Kina. *Friidrettens Trenerforening og N.F.I.F.s trener og utøver seminar.* Forelesning N.I.H. november, 1993.

25. Lydiard, A. and Gilmour, G.: *Running The Lydiard Way.* World Publications, Mountain View, California, 1978.

26. Martin, D. E. and Coe, P. N.: *Training Distance Runners.* Leisure Press. Champaign. Illonois, 1991.

27. Mc. Arthur, J.W.: Influence of body mass, body composition and exercise. In *The Gonadotropins: Basic Science and Clinical Aspects in Females.* Editors: Flamigni,C. and Givens,J. R. Serona Symposium No. 42: 203-215. Academic Press, New York, 1982.

28. Møller, K.: Slik trente Grete som baneløper. *Friidrett,* nr. 9, september, 1985a.

29. Møller, K.: Systematisering av treningen til Grete Waitz. *Upublisert materiale.* 1985b.

30. Noakes, T.: *Lore of running.* Oxford University Press, Cape Town, 1986.

31. Nurmekivi, A.: Specifisity and Individuality in Distance Running Training. *Modern Athlete and Coach,* Vol. 24, No.4, October, 1986.

32. Nurmekivi, A.: Some Basic Factors of Endurance Training in a Nuttshell, in: *Long Distances.* Contemporary Theory, Technique and Training. Edited by Jarver, J. Tafnews Press: 83-86, 1995.

33. Pisuke, A.: Planning of Endurance Training. *Modern athlete and coach.* (Athelstone, Aust.) Vol. 22. No 1., 1984.

34. Pisuke, A. and Nurmekivi, A.: Classification of Distance Running Training Methods, in *Long Distances,* editor: Jarver, J. Tafnews Press: 55-58, 1989.

35. Pisuke, A. and Nurmekivi, A.: Middle Distance Running Training Metods, in *Middle Distances. Contemporary Theory, Technique and Training.* Edited by Jarver, J. Tafnews Press: 67-70, 1991.

36. Schwarts, B., Cumming, D.C., Riordan, E., Selye, M., Yen, S.S.C. and Rebar, R.W.: Exercise-induced amenorrhea: a distinct entity? *American Journal of Obstetrics and Gynecology* 141: 662-670, 1981.

37. Shangold, M.M.: Sports and menstrual function. *Physician and Sportsmedicine* 8 (August): 66-71, 1980.

38. Skah, K.: Long Distance Training in Marokko. *Coach Conferance.* Norges idrettshøgskole, Oslo, November 9th, 1997.

39. Steffney, M.: The Training of a 10000 m Runner. *Die Lehre der Leichtathlick,* Vol 34, No. 26, 1983.

40. Tjelta, L.I.: En kartlegging og analyse av treningen til kvinnelige eliteløpere på langdistanse, sett i sammenheng med endringer i løpshastigheten ved anaerob terskel. *Hovedfagsoppgave i idrett.* Norges idrettshøgskole, Oslo, 1996.

41. Tomten, S.: Jenter og langdistansetrening sett i relasjon til risiko for benskjørhet. *Friidrettens Trenerforening og N.F.I.F.s trener og utøver-seminar.* Forelesning N.I.H.: 11.november 1995.

42. Van Aaken, E.: *Van Aaken Method.* World Publications, Mountain View, California, 1976.

43. van Dam, B.: Considerations in the Planning of Womens Distance Running Training. *Die Lehre der Leichtathletik,* Vol. 34, No. 26, 1983.

44. van den Eynde, E.: Training of Long Distance Runners. *Die Lehre der Leichtathletik,* Vol. 34, No 22, 1983.

45. Wakat, D.K., Sweeney, K.A. and Rogol, A.D.: Reproductive system function in women cross-country runners. *Medicine and Science in Sports and Exercise* 14: 263-269, 1982.